MANAGING CHANGE AND COLLABORATION IN THE HEALTH SYSTEM

Managing Change and Collaboration in the Health System

The Paradigm Approach

Alan/Sheldon

*Harvard School
of Public Health*

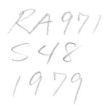

 Oelgeschlager, Gunn & Hain, Publishers, Inc.
Cambridge, Massachusetts

International Standard Book Number: 0-89946-003-8

Library of Congress Catalog Card Number: 79-19700

Printed in the United States of America

Library of Congress Cataloging in Publication Data
Sheldon, Alan, 1933-
    Managing change and collaboration in the health system.

    Includes Index.
    1. Health   facilities—Administration—Case   studies.   2. Health   facilities—
Affiliations—Case studies. 3. Health services administration—Case studies. 4. Or-
ganizational change—Case studies. 5. Interorganizational relations—Case studies.
I. Title.
RA971.S48   658'.91'3621   79-19700
ISBN 0-89946-003-8

Contents

Acknowledgments

All the studies are real—real people, real situations. Some are disguised because of the sensitivity of the situations described. The studies were conducted over the past five years, so situations reported may well have changed. To all, my grateful thanks for allowing me to study and to learn.

My grateful thanks to Susan Silverman, who gathered much of the material for the structural forms chapter and organized it as well as several of the case studies. The research work for three of the case studies was performed by Anil Gupta, who also added creatively to the concepts I have developed. To him also my gratitude. Finally, Leslie Stein has put up with me far longer than I have any right to expect; she typed and retyped superbly. I want here to express to her my appreciation and affection.

Chapter 1

Western Psychiatric Hospital

The dramatic story of a psychiatric hospital is told here. From it and another account about a clinic (Chapter 2) are drawn ideas that help illuminate some problems of organizational change and, in addition, some aspects of organizational collaboration. Several studies of collaboration are presented later.

In the late 1950s an instructor of psychiatry at a western medical school started an experimental psychotherapy program for acute psychotics at a California hospital. Initially a four-bed unit with four doctors and eight patients, in four or five years it grew to half the hospital with twenty-five doctors and seventy patients, losing along the way the founding father. The last year or so was characterized by administrative conflict with the hospital that had given them much autonomy and then later regretted it.

In this period the medical director had been joined by one of his residents, a charismatic and talented man who later became clinical director, the then medical director, and a fourth clinician. They added three more investor colleagues and set up business as a for-profit private hospital, Western Psychiatric Hospital (WPH). They sold off half their investment to a for-profit hospital company,

All the names and places in this chapter have been fictionalized.

realizing both a substantial return to the investors and a satisfactory salary to the clinicians who retained control through their seats on the board and were employed in their clinical roles via management contracts. The clinicians were not only board members, owners, and investors, but also administrators and clinicians, for each had a private practice in the hospital, and each ran a clinical unit. They did so in spite of their intention not to be a hospital. They saw themselves as more of a clan in which the chieftains of the tribe were equal, with the clinical director more equal than the others.

The hospital specialized in the treatment of severe psychotics, borderline character disorders, and sociopaths. Essentially it dealt in tertiary care, referrals from other psychiatric hospitals, and the failures of other psychiatrists. In other words, it dealt with the hardest type of patient to treat. The therapeutic technology essentially consisted of intensive psychotherapy without the aid of drugs, except on rare occasions, and without electroshock therapy. Restraints were used since the therapeutic technique was intended to break down maladaptive defenses by fostering regression. Patients were usually in the hospital from eighteen months to two years since a long period was required to break down their defenses and then to build them up.

The hospital was relatively light on administrative staff and procedures and heavy on nurses and therapeutic support staff. Under the guidance of the clinical director, it had innovated the development of a new administrative-therapeutic role, the unit leader, each responsible for part of a ward. To some degree this role had arisen in the absence of strong nursing leadership, and to some degree was a function of the particular therapy involved. Unit leaders might have backgrounds in nursing or psychology or have been attendants. They were promoted on the basis of their capacity to be effective therapeutically, and the most senior had a great deal of power in the hospital.

The hospital was originally divided into four long-term clinical wards plus an adolescent ward and an admission and evaluation ward. The three clinical owners each ran a ward. Some six of the twenty or so medical staff worked on each of the major wards and, in addition, could admit to the adolescent ward. However, no one really ran a ward, as most of the decision making was delegated and made at the ward or unit level, and the senior unit leaders, of whom there were ten, had a major say over what went on at the unit level.

Thus a unique choice of patients and an innovative form of therapy had led to the development of innovative roles and a very informal decentralized form of administration. It was clear, furthermore, that there was some self-selection for the kinds of people who found this work interesting and were good at it. Medical staff, for example, normally never had more than two to four patients, each of whom they might see for half an hour a day, five days a week. Staff tended to be somewhat compliant and, with few exceptions, busied themselves with clinical rather than administrative matters. Perhaps it was a combination of the innovative excitement and enthusiasm and the self-selected passivity that led to so many potential administrative and interpersonal conflicts being suppressed or ignored.

Success was unabated through 1975, but 1975 to 1978 proved to be a chequered and turbulent time. A private hospital, it was still heavily dependent on reimbursement of charges through insurance and Blue Cross, and the insurance organizations leaned heavily on long-term patient coverage. This resulted in a drop in referrals and therefore in census. While this was common across the United States, the specialized nature of WPH made this a particularly difficult blow. The census dropped from a maximum of 100 or so to 87 in 1976, 77 in 1977, and 70 in 1978, although the hospital is currently licensed for 100 beds and has 90 available. The hospital was able to cut back from a high of 1.9 employees per patient to 1.6, but it became clear that its unique approach was not economically viable. Coincident with these economic pressures was what appeared to be some burning out of some of the original protagonists. The then medical director withdrew entirely, although maintaining his financial interests, and the charismatic clinical director withdrew much of his energy and interest. Census pressures resulted in fewer staff and higher turnover, and those staff remaining became overburdened and with the influx of newer staff, relatively inexperienced since eighteen months to two years were required to teach people the specialized techniques. It was in response to these pressures that the hospital began to change its approach and its organization.

In 1976, in response to the economic pressures, one of the long-term wards was converted into a general psychiatry program for shorter-stay patients. The new general psychiatry program had fewer acute patients, but they were still quite sick, and there were more of them moving more rapidly through it. The three long-term wards that had had approximately seventeen beds each, although the wards were often only two thirds full, were transformed into eighteen-bed wards. The adolescent ward was essentially kept unchanged, although moved physically. The change was a difficult one, and since the clinician owners had both clinical and administrative roles on the wards, both choices and methods were questioned. Favoritism was implied, and doubts began to be raised as to whether clinical decisions might not be financially based. Medical staff worried whether there might be enough beds for their patients. They worried in spite of the fact that none of them in reality had any fewer than previously. Some of these feelings and concerns might have arisen because management was perceived as being amateur, without long-term plans and moving from crisis to crisis.

The success of the previous approach was being questioned. Whether real or imagined, conflicts once ignored or suppressed began to preoccupy the attention of the staff, and the clinical and medical directors in particular were seen to be in competition. Since the clinical director was identified in everyone's minds with the original and pure approach, while the medical director was seen to be largely responsible for the evolving new approach and heavier emphasis on administration, it is not surprising that staff ambivalence about new methods that might be required but were unwelcome would get played out on these two characters. The medical director did not diminish their concerns when he began to tighten up administrative procedures and appointed a new managerially oriented nursing director. To make matters worse, she had a background in reality therapy rather than long-term therapy.

Reaction was not long forthcoming. It was felt at all levels that excitement, intuition, and loving were being replaced by dollar signs and administration. Fewer beds and the lack of success of an ill-conceived outpatient clinic turned off the medical staff, who themselves referred fewer patients when they had any to refer. Unit leaders felt threatened by the shift to formal structures but felt despairing about what they could do since they, not incorrectly, perceived themselves to be uniquely adapted to their existing situation, and to have little hope of job transfer elsewhere. The general feeling was one of moving from a family to a business, and many incidents that once had passed without comment now raised hostilities. Money interests on the part of the once revered clinician owners were felt to be suspect. The pay inequity between unit leaders and psychiatrists was felt to be intolerable in view of the relative load taken by the unit leaders. Staff involvement diminished, morale dropped, and turnover exacerbated the problem for those that remained. More extreme symptoms included some staff themselves succumbing to psychiatric disorders and a number of suicides among discharged patients, largely from the new program and for the first time in the history of the hospital. Perhaps despair is contagious.

It was in this context that the final blow fell. After the resignation of one social worker for personal reasons, the remaining three attempted to renegotiate their relationship with the hospital. There had been a year-long background to this. Having always done therapy cases under supervision, it had been proposed that one social worker see a patient alone. The physicians had responded sharply, whether the issue was economic or territorial, and had banned this process. Believing, not incorrectly, that the hospital was making a lot of money on them and fed up with working a fifty-hour week for a forty-hour salary and then even longer hours if they wished to see their private patients, the social workers asked for a better split of the clinical fee plus higher payment for their administrative services. Alternatively, they asked that they have a relationship like the medical staff in which they worked on contract using the hospital premises when appropriate. The social workers knew largely what they wanted. But both sides were inexperienced in negotiating, and what was felt to be a condescending attitude on the part of the clinician owners who handled the negotiation, led to what the social workers felt was a totally inadequate response that resulted in all three resigning.

The picture, in fact, while bleak, was not as desperate as many felt. What is revealed is two worlds in conflict. The first world had evolved with perfect fit between its parts but had begun to find its success in the larger world diminishing. Perhaps because of the perfect fit between its parts, it was unwilling or unable to make those adjustments that might have helped it repair its economic distress. The clinical director had once said that they never wanted a hospital but felt themselves to be a clan. Now the clan members would rather fight (or have the institution die) than switch. Entrapped in their own world view, they not only could not make changes that could keep them alive because it meant to them a betrayal of an ideal but they could not let the remainder of the organization do it for them either. As the medical director began to be identified with the development of an alternative world, he and it were undercut in two disastrous ways. The new world was put down by old-timers as involving a more superficial form of therapy, and the new therapy could not be carried out with the old staff. Short-term therapy for less sick people cannot be approached using the same techniques and staff as long-term therapy for very sick people, because it must be defence enhancing, not defence reducing. There is no time to break and rebuild, so aftercare support is required. The war between these two worlds is what Thomas Kuhn calls "paradigmatic conflict" (see Chapter 3).

Suffice it to say that the simple understanding that two totally different worlds were engaged in a brutal and bruising fight led to the beginning of an appreciation of how to approach the solution.

Remedy lay at a number of levels, but first and most important was the separation of the two paradigms that were warring. It was proposed that the hospital be divided into two divisions—physically, organizationally, and fiscally. Different people should be in charge of each, and there should even be two nursing directors. Different staff should work on each with newly recruited staff working on the general psychiatry program. Administrative rules, procedures, and organizations would be more structured and formal on the general psychiatry program, and traditionally informal on the long-term units. The basic failure was in not recognizing that what they were engaged in was paradigmatic change. In other words, they had attempted to change only one dimension of the organization, namely, the kind of patients they were treating, without recognizing that what they were doing really meant changing many dimensions of the organization simultaneously. Apparently, this simple model helped, and in the ensuing months, the divisional concept was implemented and even symbolized by having the general psychiatry program staff wear uniforms as a sign of their greater formality. Turnover dropped, morale rose, and, Phoenix-like, what may have seemed terminal became a new beginning.

Chapter 2

The South Clinic

The South Clinic is a medical group practice organized as a partnership. Eighty-five physicians are partners, and seven of them are on a board of management. Under the board is a medical director, an associate and an assistant medical director, and an administrative staff. It employs many other doctors in addition to the partners, and it has a total of 650 employees. The partnership rents the clinic building from the South Medical Foundation, and the partners and staff use the Foundation Hospital.

The South Medical Foundation is a nonprofit corporation that has several operating divisions. These include the Foundation Hospital (with 1869 employees), the Graduate Medical Education Division, the School of Allied Health Sciences, and the Research Institute. Additional divisions of the foundation include finance, employee relations, planning and development, and public affairs. There is, in addition, a service corporation whose stock is held solely by people who work at the medical institutions. This corporation owns and operates a hotel and affiliated services. The president of the foundation is also chief executive officer of the hospital (a recent innovation), and there is a fifty-one-member board of trustees. An executive committee has fifteen members, seven of whom are both

All the names and places in this chapter have been fictionalized.

physicians and partners in the clinic. Not counting the hospital employees, there are 107 employees of the foundation.

INTRODUCTION

The South Clinic started in 1940 when five professors at a southern school of medicine in surgery, urology, otolaryngology, gynecology, and orthopedics decided that a well-organized group practice would meet a great medical need in the area. Advice was sought from existing clinics such as Lahey, Mayo, Minnesota, and Cleveland. Suggestions included seeking a location permitting greater expansion than might currently be envisaged, referring patients to hospitals operated by others so that the professors would not have to run a hospital themselves, and resigning their medical school appointments so that they could devote themselves full time to clinic practice. Financial assistance from philanthropists was sought, initially fruitlessly. Finally, a patient who ran a bank proffered his bank's support should plans be forthcoming.

An office building was found. A first public announcement mentioned "plans for establishment of a 'little Mayo Clinic' where people from all over the south and from South and Central American countries could come for diagnostic checkups by groups of the most skilled medical specialists in the city . . . ." It is noteworthy that the market for the clinic has not changed in four decades.

The notice that the first building was to be purchased started many rumors among local physicians, most of whom were bitterly opposed to group practice, feeling it was unfair competition. On Holy Thursday night of that year, anonymous people sent each of the five founders a small leather bag containing thirty silver dimes and a typewritten note that read, "to help pay for your clinic, from the local physicians, surgeons and dentists." The implication that the founders were Judases did not change their plans.

The original five partners agreed that each was to invest an equal portion of the capital and operating funds and receive an equal share of the earnings. The South Clinic opened its doors to patients on January 2, 1942. The first patients who came represented primarily consolidated clientele of the founders. Appointments were arranged through a central appointment office, records were filed in a central record room, and reports were filed in the patients' records. Clinical x-ray labs and the pharmacy were centralized. Bookkeeping and accounting were also centralized, and patients received a single statement for all services rendered. Physicians hospitalized patients at a local infirmary under the care of the clinic staff. Soon patients were being referred to the clinic for complete service—that is, for a diagnostic survey or clinic check—rather than for care by a particular physician.

The foundation soon added laymen to the board of trustees. These new members were competent businessmen who could help in the handling of business affairs. In addition, the foundation considered changing the partnership into an association similar to Mayo or into a foundation like Cleveland or Ford, but state laws prohibited the practice by a nonprofit corporation or foundation, so the partnership was retained. However, in 1944 the Medical Foundation was created by dissolving the property-holding corporation and giving its assets to the nonprofit corporation. Henceforth the clinic leased its buildings, grounds, furnishings, and equipment from the foundation, which applied the rentals to its declared purposes of education, research, and charity. The Mayo's foundation was similar in that it ensured the continued success of the clinic after the founders died. Today the foundation continues this tradition.

The critical shortage of hospital beds in the city forced the clinic to consider either developing its own hospital or joining the university. Clearly there was a need for a new hospital of about 300 beds but the foundation trustees, while appreciating the need, felt unable to raise the funds, although they offered to operate the proposed hospital and absorb deficits. Federal funds being lacking, the proposition languished while the clinic continued to expand. The infirmary was asked for an additional wing, but could not manage the financing without the university's aid. It was not until late in 1946 that, after many difficulties, the trustees were able to obtain an ex-army hospital; in 1947 the Foundation Hospital finally opened.

The clinic soon required more hospital beds, but neither the infirmary nor the university could (or would) respond, and so the foundation eventually raised the money directly. In 1951 they bought from the local railroad a site consisting of twenty-one acres lying between a major highway and a river. It was on this site that first the hotel—dedicated to patients, families, and visitors—and then the hospital (1954) and the clinic were built. In 1957 much of the clinic moved to some floors of the hotel, and in 1959 the research building was completed. The new clinic building was started in 1961 and completed in 1963.

The South Medical Institutions went through three organizational phases.

THE FOUNDERS' ERA, 1941-LATE 1950s

The Founders' Era is characterized by having the decision making in the hands of the five founders at multiple levels.

South Clinic: During this period the clinic was a partnership composed solely of the five founders. The founders headed the major departments, and the other physicians were employees of the partnership. The board of management at the South Clinic was formed at the behest of the employed physicians. It was composed of the five founders plus two senior employed physicians, the chief of medicine, and the associate chief of surgery. The chief of medicine also served on the board of management with them. The first two medical directors were recruited from academia. Their performances proved unsatisfactory so one founder agreed to lend stability to the group practice by becoming the medical director. In addition, a less than satisfactory business manager was replaced early in the history of the organizations by a strong director, who remains in this position today.

The Foundation: The board of trustees of the foundation comprised the five founders plus two strong lay trustees. The original founder served as president of the foundation, but the role of the president was largely titular. The hospital director's post was filled, after the hospital was established, by relatively undistinguished individuals at first.

THE SUCCESSORS' ERA, LATE 1950s-EARLY 1970s

The Successors' Era was characterized by replacement of the founders in all of their multiple roles by a group of hand-picked successors.

The South Clinic: The partnership was broadened in 1957 by formation of a new partnership. Half of the ownership remained in the hands of the five founders, the remaining half belonging to a new group of physicians eligible on the basis of five years of service. Provision was made to phase out the original founding partners over a number of years.

The five founders on the board of management were gradually replaced by senior physicians, usually department heads. Members of the board served ten-year terms and were eligible to succeed themselves and to serve until age sixty-five. Any vacancy would be filled by the board of management, and the partnership could reject the proposed candidate only by a vote of 75 percent. In general, the board of management was composed of major department or division heads. One of the founders stepped down from the medical director position in his seventies. He was succeeded by a physician who had served as the associate medical director and who had headed the department of colon and rectal surgery. There was a subtle change in the role of the medical director during this period of time. While the former was one of five founders, the latter became the *primum inter pares*. He headed the board of management, the finance committee, and other important decision-making bodies. The director took on the additional role of the administrative director of the South Medical Foundation.

The Foundation: The two original laymen on the board of trustees were succeeded by two other powerful figures from the business community. The founders were gradually replaced during this period of time by the members of the board of management. The new medical director succeeded the original founder as president of the South Medical Foundation and at the same time assumed the title of chief executive officer of the South Medical Center. The position of hospital director was filled after 1960 by an administrator who was hampered by ill health in the last years of his service. A board of governors of the South Foundation Hospital had been formed after the current hospital was constructed, but it had a largely titular and honorary function. The original members of the board of governors were serving largely in recognition of their role as donors to the foundation and to the hospital. They were replaced gradually by an energetic group of young businessmen who felt isolated from the decision-making process since this role was filled by the board of trustees.

CURRENT ERA, EARLY 1970s TO PRESENT

The South Clinic: The partnership was characterized by some change. The eligibility for election to the partnership was reduced to three years' service. There are now eighty-five partners. The value of the partnership, which was approximately $2500 when the expanded partnership was formed in 1957, now exceeds $100,000. There is some subtle undercurrent of sentiment to restrict entry into the partnership to avoid diluting the holdings of the current partners.

The partnership agreement was rewritten in the early 1970s to provide popular election to the board of management. Annually the partnership has two candidates presented to it, and the majority vote determines the winner. Members elected to the board of management serve seven-year terms and cannot succeed themselves. The initial phases of popular election brought a subtle change in character to the board. The most visible and most vocal antiestablishment candidates tended to be elected. Only one department head is on the board of management at the present time. In general, as the major department heads have relinquished administrative roles, they have not been replaced by members of the board of management. Recruiting from outside plus a tendency to identify talent early has resulted in the fact that in recent years anywhere from four to six major departments have been headed by physicians who are not yet partners in the group practice. The second medical director gave up his role with the South Medical Foundation and was succeeded in 1975 by a younger physician.

The Foundation: Largely to address concerns that the role of the hospital board of governors was hollow, there was a drastic change in the board of trustees in the early 1970s. A very large board of trustees was created with over forty members, incorporating members of the previous board of trustees, the board of governors, others from the South Clinic and the community, and physicians from the South Clinic. As the decision-making body of the foundation, an executive committee composed of eight laymen and seven physicians from the board of trustees was created. The seven physicians had served on the board of trustees in the previous era so that as time passed, they were phased out of their administrative roles when they reached the age of sixty, and they were removed from the board of management of the clinic by a change in the election rules. The physicians on the executive committee were former department heads and former members of the board of management.

In the early 1970s the illness and subsequent death of the hospital administrator mandated a search for a replacement. The lay members on the search committee became convinced that they would be unable to recruit a man of stature without making him head of the foundation as well. Such a person was recruited and became, in the autumn of 1974, president and chief executive officer of the South Medical Foundation. The second medical director—who until that time had been president of the South Medical Foundation, medical director of the South Clinic, and chief executive officer of the South Medical Center—became the chairman of the board of trustees.

Thus the situation in the mid-1970s was fraught with the potential for miscommunication and polarization between groups, entirely independent of the personalities involved. There were three identifiable groups of physicians in the power structure: (1) the board of management and medical director; (2) the major department heads who carry line responsibility for running the departments, carrying out the mandates of the board of management, and (3) the physician members of the executive committee of the South Medical Foundation. In contrast to previous times in which the same group of physicians constituted all three groups, there had now become practically no overlap between the three groups.

There was a legacy of mistrust between the physicians of the clinic and the foundation. The clinic had given the local medical school a large donation at a time when merger seemed possible, and continued to give the foundation money even in lean years. The foundation, as the clinic's landlord, increased its rent threefold from a low of about $350,000 a year.

Some of the interorganizational difficulties seemed to be rooted in the personalities of the various individuals. The new chief executive officer (CEO) proved to be an able administrator, but he developed heavy insulation from the line activities of the foundation. After his arrival, in rapid order he recruited and hired a hospital administrator, a personnel manager, a public relations director, and an array of other administrators whom he clustered into his management executive committee. Some problems arose when a member of the management executive committee was performing functions for the clinic as well as the foundation. The clinic would be charged a pro rata share of the cost of operating a division such as public relations at a time when the division chief was a member of the management executive committee and directly answerable to the foundation CEO. This new CEO's style did not mesh well with the views of some of the more conservative members of the medical staff. He was dedicated to making his mark as a health care administrator and tended to view the new frontiers of health care administration as lying in the formation of multihospital conglomerates.

Starting in 1976, a variety of hospital affiliations, takeovers, or amalgamations were considered. These proposals involved an ear, nose, and throat hospital that eventually came under the foundation banner, a hospital in an adjacent city that was having a trying time, a new private hospital and group practice in Latin America, and a children's hospital, that had not only census but cash-flow and managerial problems as well. While these latter three hospitals were not acquired for a variety of reasons, with each succeeding venture there seemed to be a flood of publicity and community reaction, some of it adverse. A local periodical ran an extensive story under the title "The South Octopus." At the same time that all of this was going on, negotiations were completed with the state for supplying house staff to the newest member of the state's charity hospital system, which provided training for South Clinic junior staff and helped out the state, too.

During the discussions about these hospital affiliations, it became clear that the aspirations and desires of clinic management and foundation management were not congruent. The management of the group practice tended to view such ventures as desirable to the extent that they furthered the success of the group practice, while foundation management tended to view all acquisitions as desirable whether the group practice was involved or not. Often the acquisition would have to involve the addition of a new group of nonclinic physicians who would then need to relate to the foundation. By early 1978 there appeared to be a progressive polarization between the board of management and the partnership of the South Clinic on the one hand, and the management and to a lesser extent the board of trustees of the South Medical Foundation on the other. The clinic medical director attempted to serve as a buffer between these two groups, but it became apparent that further severe deterioration left a serious question as to whether the clinic board of management would be willing to engage in any joint projects with the South Medical Foundation. It was at this point that the foundation CEO was confronted with the fact that physicians' confidence in him had eroded to a point of no return, and he resigned.

While the relationships between the clinic and the foundation were deteriorating, the rationale for keeping them separate seemed to be diminishing. As the management of the foundation and its hospital strengthened, it seemed less and less efficient to duplicate many of the administrative departments. Strengthening the board of lay trustees had led paradoxically to an increase in their frustration as they found themselves unable to have much effective influence over the somewhat mysterious and paramount workings of the doctor-dominated clinic.

SUMMARY

Over its fifty years, the clinic has continued to grow and succeed. This achievement has come in spite of, perhaps rather than because of, a decision-making process that has largely been one of reacting to events as they impressed themselves rather than one of initiating actions.

The institution is now in the third generation of its "family," leaning toward professional management for the first time, as demonstrated by the hiring of the new CEO. In the first generation the clinic was managed essentially by the founders and then by their successors. The third generation seems to recognize the need to share with professional managers the running of the institution, or to become managers themselves. However, the CEO's evident skills and energy were mitigated by his lack of involvement with the physicians who dominated the power structure and who regarded his actions as opportunistic rather than strategic.

Finally, for the first five decades of its existence, the South Clinic was essentially the only institution in the city, and perhaps in the region, where the first-rate physician who did not wish to go into private practice would care to practice. Today the first-rate physician has many alternatives, including better opportunities for private practice, as well as teaching hospitals, medical schools, and community hospitals, where he may feel that he can get a higher salary, greater freedom, or more organizational support for his ambitions than the South Clinic offers.

SYMPTOMS OF FRUSTRATION

The conflict, a certain degree of which is appropriate for any organization, had obviously risen to an abrasive and dysfunctional level. In addition, concern was being expressed by some partners and administrators over the present or future likelihood of some erosion of the market as well as an increase in the turnover of physicians. It was noted also that in the South Clinic fewer doctors than before were leaders in their fields.

Some felt that many of the recent problems and the breakdown in communication was attributable to personalities, and that they would be remedied by the CEO's departure. Others felt that while personalities may have contributed, there were more fundamental problems affecting the clinic and the hospital. Doing nothing was possible, but that risked the institutions' future options being preempted by others. What really was wrong, and what really needed doing?

SOME QUESTIONS: THE TWO PARADIGMS ELUCIDATED

The environment in which the institution was operating had changed markedly in recent years. It had become more complex and more competitive, and in addition, of course, the organization had grown to a size that could not be managed easily or in the informal fashion that was possible in earlier days. Attitudes and values, however, had not changed as sharply, and the old remained intermixed with the new.

Traditional physician ambivalence about management in particular and leadership in general—which has often led doctors to find it easier to say no than yes, especially by default—had led to their reluctance to either take on management responsibilities or delegate them fully to others. Certainly, physicians exercised power, but the institution had not been "managed" in the usual sense of that word. This ambivalence was now frustrating lay trustees, and their tolerance was diminishing. It also discouraged excellence in lay administration. This ambivalence resulted in a situation in which there was some feeling that the department chiefs were the most important roles for the future of the organization, and yet despite this responsibility, they were given negligible power. The board of management, representing the partnership, made policy (to the extent that it was made) and managed, which included hiring, firing, setting salaries, appointing department and section chiefs, and establishing departmental budgets. The question was, did the doctors want the institution to be managed? Or did they want to manage it themselves?

There was clearly some consensus that the clinic was an organizational setting in which physicians could participate free of many constraints that they believed they would experience in other settings. It was more supportive than private practice while less constraining than a medical school. However, there were many different views as to what additional constraints would be acceptable if required and in what direction they should go. Thus the identity was inchoate, which was beneficial, since possibly disruptive differences could be contained in an illusion of unanimity. However, the institution was not proceeding in any defined direction with a consequent set of clear-cut actions and decisions. The cost of clarifying its identity might be the loss of some people or support; the cost of not doing so would be a diminished institution. The question was, did the partnership and the boards wish to clarify identity and therefore strategy, decision, and action?

In the governance of the institution, distinctions among influencing, policy making, and managing had become blurred. The board of management made policy and certainly managed. The partnership felt that it should not only influence but should also make policy. The managers (the medical director and the department heads, for example) felt that they were not being allowed to manage. As a result, policies were not being made and managing was not being done as effectively as it might have been. In an expansive era that could contain some slippage, this was not perhaps crucial. The question was whether these three important functions should be clearly identified and separated, as, for example, that the partnership should influence the selection of those it elects, and that once elected, the board should make policy and should appoint those whom it wishes to manage and leave them to do that.

In any organization there is always a dilemma of what information to share as well as with whom. People always want more information, often meaning more influence, but when they get it, whether it be in the form of memoranda or meetings, they resent the time it takes. Power in any organization can to some degree be exercised by the sharing or withholding of information. At this point in the life of the South Clinic, there seemed to be many rumors, fantasies, and misapprehensions, especially between the foundation and the clinic, due to a lack of information. The question was whether the institution wished to disclose information about relevant matters more fully or not.

The increase in turnover among physicians had been noted. It had been pointed out that there were attractive options both in private practice, which offered higher incomes, and in teaching institutions, which offered organizational support. Some felt that it was important to stabilize the physician population. The question was whether South was prepared to accept a higher degree of turnover as a fact of life of the institution, or wished to alter its organizational environment so as to make it more attractive for young physicians to come and to stay.

For historical and tax-related reasons, the clinic and the foundation were created as separate entities. Although once essentially governed as a single entity, the distance between them had grown.

This had led to communication and governance problems, as well as to inefficiencies. The question was whether the two institutions at some future point should become better joined so that they could be better managed or whether they should remain as essentially separate entities.

The failure to confront some of the preceding questions had led to a mild condition of doublethink. On the one hand, some said that the department chiefs were all important; the same people, however, also said that the department chiefs had sufficient power, when in fact they had little if any. People believed that there was a unanimous view of their institutional identity, yet it was anything but unanimous. The advantage of doublethink is that it maintains the illusion of oneness; the disadvantage is that it results in potentially difficult consequences when decisions are not followed through. The question was whether the institution wished to confront its differences and the consequences of its desires, or wished to maintain its illusions.

The institution is typical of many physician-dominated institutions in that its solutions to problems were somewhat short run and piecemeal. This approach is understandable to some degree since most physicians' tasks are relatively short run. However, the organizational problems that faced the institution could be dealt with only in a long-run and fundamental fashion, not in a piecemeal one. The question was, did the institution wish to deal with fundamental and long-run issues, or did it wish to continue to muddle through on a short-run and piecemeal basis?

These questions or dilemmas could be summarized as a conflict between personal values and philosophies facing organizational imperatives and realities with distinct consequences. The issue was whether a traditional approach, which had certainly been successful in the past, of muddling through, should become more deliberative, and whether the variety of views and concomitant differences that characterize any vital organization should be clouded or should be confronted and lead to clear-cut choices.

The two paradigms thus elucidated were those of *physician muddling through* versus *deliberative management*. The latter required not only attitude and value change but a different kind of person in the managerial role (especially if physician) and a different organizational power and decision-making structure, probably one cutting across the institutions in some fashion. The ultimate organizational form might well be a matrix in which there would be some functions totally centralized for both institutions and some departments decentralized within each institution but reporting both to the institutions (for responsiveness) and to a central department head (for efficiency). In turn, this organizational structural change would require some shift in the ownership of the clinic, perhaps from a partnership into a corporation. These changes represent a transformation of paradigm as well as an emergence of a true "supraparadigm" in a single central identity for the organization transcending but containing the separate existing identities. These changes contrast with the side-by-side emergence of new paradigm in the example of Western Psychiatric Hospital. Given the need to change a total way of operation, the first and hardest change is one of attitude. This process requires much time and some replacing of people if they cannot themselves change. It also requires a transitional process in which existing members of the organization have confidence. Thus it was proposed that before any major structural changes were considered, the following actions be considered. These actions were felt to be realistic given existing constraints in the form of attitudes, and given the goal of transforming those attitudes, which when achieved would then allow further consideration of future strategy and organization, too threatening to deal with presently.

Two new and cross-institutional bodies were created to deliberate and enact policy concerning the total institution. The first, a joint policy committee, would consist of the board of management together with the executive committee of the board of trustees. The second, a joint operating committee, would bring together the clinic medical director and his associate and the major department and division heads in the clinic, the hospital, and the foundation.

The reason for the interim and possibly lengthy bridging process was that the ultimate state proposed represented a paradigmatic shift that would be totally unacceptable to the existing clinic organization. Time must pass, attitudes changed, and information and education be shared in order to reach that different state of being.

Chapter 3

Paradigms in Change and Collaboration

PARADIGM

The two preceding case studies introduced the concept of "paradigm." A decade ago Thomas Kuhn shocked the scientific world with his analysis of the development of scientific theory, in which he suggested that science advanced through evolutionary and revolutionary periods.[1] Most science, what he calls "normal science," works within an accepted set of rules and spends its time exploring the nooks and crannies of them. Occasionally there comes along a kind of science that changes the rules, which he calls "paradigmatic science." A paradigm is a scientific theory and also more than that. It is what the members of a scientific community share; and conversely, a scientific community consists of people who share a paradigm. It is both a way of going about the business of science as well as what the scientist sees. Paradigms are, in a way, worlds as well as world views. People can agree on identifying a paradigm without being able to agree on exactly what it is; in other words, it is a useful vague term.

Paradigms guide science and scientific research by providing models as well as rules. Normal science can get along without rules as long as scientists accept the way in which things are done. Rules become important when paradigms or models are felt to be in question. So the period just before a paradigm changes is marked by intense argument over whether models and rules are proper or not. Such debates intensify with the appearance of a paradigm, i.e., a new and alternative world and world view.

Crises are prerequisites for the emergence of new theories. When scientists find that old theories don't altogether work anymore, they may begin to lose faith in them and consider alternatives, but they do not give up on them. In fact, scientists discard theories only if an alternative theory is available to take its place. So the decision to reject one paradigm is always simultaneously the decision to accept another. Crises therefore loosen stereotypes and provide the additional evidence that helps facilitate a fundamental paradigm shift. The problem with arguing about paradigms is that each group uses its own to argue in that paradigm's defense. Because paradigms represent totally different worlds and world views, arguments cannot be logical since the basic assumptions of either party are totally different and not shared. Values are so different that the proponents of competing paradigms are always at least slightly at cross-purposes and are bound partly to talk past each other. Though each may hope to convert the other to his way of seeing and to sharing his paradigm, neither may hope to prove the case. The competition between paradigms is not the sort of battle that can be resolved by proofs, for the proponents of competing paradigms will often disagree even about the list of problems that any candidate for a paradigm must resolve. In other words, they not only live in different worlds, they see different worlds out there even though the objects are the same.

When they have adopted a new paradigm, scientists then use new instruments and look in new places. In other words, they see a different world with their own new internal world. It is as though the professional community sharing the new paradigm were suddenly transported to another planet where familiar objects are seen in a different light and are joined by unfamiliar ones as well. After such a revolution, scientists are responding to a different world: "What were ducks in the scientists' world before the revolution are rabbits after." Since new paradigms are born from old, old terms, concepts, and approaches fall into new relationships in a new paradigm, and the inevitable result is some kind of misunderstanding between the two competing schools. The proponents of competing paradigms practice their trades in different worlds and see different things when they look from the same point in the same direction. Both look at the external world, and what they look at has not changed, but they see different things and see them in different relations, one to the other. So before they can hope to communicate fully, one group or the other must experience the conversion that might be called "paradigm shift." Just because it is a transition between different worlds, this transition cannot be made a step at a time but must occur all at once, although not necessarily instantaneously, or not at all. How can this transposition be made? Scientists, being only human, cannot always admit their errors, even when confronted with strict proof; thus the shift from an old to a new paradigm is not based totally on logic. The shift of allegiance is a conversion experience that cannot be forced. Lifelong resistance to such a change is not to be unexpected, particularly from those whose productive careers have been committed to an older tradition of normal science. Such an investment may produce not only intense allegiance but intense antipathy to any threatened change.

The source of resistance is the assurance that the older paradigm will ultimately solve all its problems, that nature can be shoved into the box that the paradigm provides. Inevitably, at times of revolution, that assurance seems stubborn and pigheaded, as indeed it sometimes becomes. But it should be remembered that it is through normal science that the professional community of scientists fully explores the value of the older paradigm and discovers those shortcomings that paradoxically then begin to create the need for a new one.

To say that resistance is inevitable and legitimate, and that change cannot be justified by proof, is not to say that no arguments are relevant or that scientists cannot be persuaded to change their minds. A generation may be required to effect change, but scientific communities have again and again been converted to new paradigms. These conversions occur in spite of indefinite resistance on the part of older and more experienced scientists because many scientists can be reached one way or another. Conversions occur a few at a time until, after the last holdouts have died, the whole profession once again practices under a single but now different paradigm. How does such conversion occur? Or posed differently, not how can we convert one or another individual, but what are the dynamics of the community that sooner or later re-forms as a single group? The arguments for change are based initially on the proposition that the new paradigm can solve the problems that have led the old one into crisis. These arguments may not be compelling. New paradigms may be advanced as being neater, more suitable, or simpler than the old, and these esthetic considerations can sometimes be decisive. Finally, there are two other elements of a paradigm that are powerful and persuasive: beliefs and values. Beliefs in particular models are shared by groups of scientists. They supply the group with acceptable analogies and metaphors and thus help to determine what will be accepted and what will not. Values are shared even more widely, and their particular importance emerges at crisis times when choices have to be made.

ORGANIZATIONAL PARADIGM

The contention of this book is that organizations work according to paradigms, as the case studies suggest and Kuhn's words describe. An organization is a world with a particular view out that colors what its members see and let in. That organizational world consists of what organizational theorists have described extensively. People practicing their technologies are organized by their tasks and structured into relationships kept dynamic by the way they are measured and controlled. All this is directed toward some end, called "purpose" or "strategy," sometimes explicit, sometimes implicit. Inevitably, these people are to some degree self-selected, inadvertently or deliberately, and share values and attitudes.

Theory (for example, see Lawrence and Lorsch[2]), especially contingency theory, would have it that any organization not actually failing must have some degree of fit both among the dimensions of technology, structure, people, and control system and between them and the environment. Fit is rarely perfect, so organizations constantly tinker with some dimension—what might be called "normal change." Normal change, being experienced as a need to tune up, is rarely resisted strenuously and often may be needed when the environment (the market, resources) shifts in some unstabilizing fashion.

But all organizations tend toward a paradigm—toward some perfect fit and some (idealized) way of working that is cherished. Normal change does not normally threaten that paradigm. Occasionally there is a perfect fit when all dimensions are harmoniously directed toward some cherished end. At that point the organization becomes ultrastable and an end in itself. Any change, in any dimension, now threatens the paradigm; the world will dissolve if any part of it changes. If anything is lost, all is lost. Western Psychiatric Hospital reached that point. It is then that people feel they would rather fight (or die) than change.

Ackoff and Emery have defined "adaptiveness" as the ability of a system to modify itself or its environment when either has changed to the system's disadvantage so as to regain at least some of its lost efficiency.[3] The process of normal change is the organization being adaptive. It is also called "organizational learning," for as the organization gets information about what is less than adaptive, it does something about it. Organizations with perfect fit are in a paradigmatic or ultrastable state and are unable to be adaptive or to learn. Because changing any dimension is threatening, they can change none. The normal organization is open to learning and therefore functions as an open system. The organization in a paradigmatic state functions as a closed system, for any information entering it about its failure has to be rejected because of what it implies. It is for this reason that an organization in this state begins to act as though the paradigm were an end rather than a means to the mission of the organization. Keeping who we are and what we do is more important than whether this has value in and to the outside world. Moreover, if the process of normal change becomes extensive enough to threaten the paradigm, it too will be resisted, and the organization will start to behave as though it were ultrastable.

Change under these circumstances can be only discontinuous, and never continuous as it can in normal change. The organization changes not at all for a while and then if the fit between the organization and the environment is poor enough, the old paradigm must be renounced and a new one adopted, and there is a lurch to a new, relatively steady state. It is for this reason that questions must be raised about the possibility of designing truly learning organizations. Since learning is usually regarded as a continuous process, it is clear from this argument that not all organizations at all times can in fact learn continuously. An organization is not unlike a crystal that settles down into a stable state but, under changes of pressure, shifts radically to a new stable state.

PARADIGMATIC RESISTANCES AND CONDITIONS

What are some of the characteristics of adherence to paradigms that produce resistance and the causes that need to be tackled if change is to be brought about?

The closed paradigmatic state is not unlike the state of groupthink described by Irving Janis.[4] Members of the organization collude to avoid any questioning of their ideology or what they do. They seem to enter a state of doublethink, in which they simultaneously acknowledge and deny aspects of the organization that do not work. Thus, at the South Clinic, doctors said they felt the department chairman's role was perfectly viable yet acknowledged that the chairman had no power to affect anything. There is an illusion of unanimity in which people repeatedly make statements that they believe are shared by others, yet they never actually check them out. Finally, any deviance is regarded as betrayal or desertion. One of the reasons that organizations in such states are hard to change is that there is a bundling process in which all the dimensions of the organization are regarded as crucial to one another, and any threatened change in one threatens the whole. Normal change techniques cannot work under these circumstances. Normal change techniques involve a large measure of rationality. Kuhn points out, and these studies echo his, that paradigm change is only partly rational.

The need for a paradigmatic change or shift comes about under two circumstances. One, if an organization enters a paradigmatic state, it becomes closed and stops adapting. At some point it will get out of fit with its environment, and when this becomes significant enough, a paradigmatic shift must occur. More commonly, paradigmatic shifts occur when a changing factor to which the organization has been responding adaptively and normally reaches a point that requires multidimensional adaptation on the part of the organization. In other words, normal change is a change in one dimension. Paradigmatic change is a change in several or all dimensions at once. Often what may happen is that an organization will go on behaving as though normal change will do when in fact there is a need for a paradigmatic shift. One may often see organizations squirming, changing this dimension or that, yet finding no significant and effective result. There is a tinkering with the structure or a fiddling with a job definition, yet what is needed is a change of the whole.

It is for this reason that techniques appropriate to dealing with normal change are not at all appropriate to dealing with paradigmatic change. Being open, confronting, involving, and working through resistances where they occur are all reasonable and appropriate ways of dealing with normal change where resistances are not enormous and worlds are not being shattered. Paradigmatic change involves a radical change in world and world view. Often the old world is felt to be dying, and there is a mourning to be experienced. If a new paradigm exists, it may be hated and abhorred as in Western Psychiatric Hospital. If none exists, a known old world, however fallible, is to be replaced by the unknown. Thus it is hardly surprising that such a major upheaval requires special handling. But even prior to managing these emotional volcanoes is the need to establish, far more radically than in normal change, the death of the old paradigm, for as long as it lingers, the new one will have little hope for survival.

PARADIGMATIC
CHANGE: APPROACHES

Too much change is overwhelming. Given that paradigmatic shifts involve multidimensional changes and that people have to be anchored in stability and security in order to entertain change without becoming unhinged, the change process must be sequenced and modulated.

It should start, like any, with a diagnosis, but one that questions not only the effectiveness of the existing way of doing things but the world and beliefs of the members of the organization. As in the South Clinic example, it may be possible to identify the existing paradigm and to raise questions about its shortcomings. Only if there is sufficient concern with the lack of success of the existing paradigm will an exploration of alternative new ones become possible. It is but later in the process that one may begin to identify and lay out alternative new paradigms and subsequently redesign the organization when a choice has been made. This questioning process, in which the organization is confronted with whether it wishes to stay the same (and face the consequences) or change, may also tackle the bundling phenomenon and facilitate the unlinking of factors so that irrational connections can be weakened. A second crucial element is the identification of values and beliefs, especially those that are contributing to the problem and those that may hinder or facilitate movement toward a solution. As Kuhn points out, the three keys to paradigm death and rebirth are the efficacy of the new paradigm (and sterility of the old) and the values and beliefs of the organization's members.

The two case studies represent, in microcosm, the three types of paradigmatic shift: (1) side by side, (2) transformation, and (3) supraparadigm.

1. *Side by side.* In Western Psychiatric Hospital the new paradigm emerges alongside the old, which continues to exist. The prerequisite for successful change is the buffering—physically, organizationally, and fiscally—of each from the other. The hospital's failure to do so led to a turbulent and bitter struggle.

2. *Transformation.* In the South Clinic (and later in Newbury) we see elements of transformation and supraparadigm, mostly the former. Transformation is lengthy, and value and belief change are crucial predecessors of any later structural changes, as is repudiation of the old paradigm. The new cannot be entertained until the old is moribund if not defunct. This requires:

a. Condemnation through a careful process of confronting consequences. The old may need a push through neglect of normal
change before a shift is entertained.
b. Attitude change through presentation of data and, if necessary,
changing people in critical roles.
c. A transitional organization in which steps a and b may be
accomplished and which, since it will replace the old before the
new is there to be experienced, must be a process and structure
that is trusted.
d. A mourning process for what is gone.

3. *Supraparadigm.* In purest form, the supraparadigm is the concept of Europe as put forward by Jean Monnet. It contains, but
transcends, the old paradigms. It must offer a positive vision (rather
than, as in side by side and transformation, something to replace
something else that does not work).

Finally, it is probably true that all three types of change are
distinctly helped by the existence of a leader who transcends the
warring or failing paradigms and is not identified with one side or
another except, as in the last case, with something above all.

WHY COLLABORATE?

The argument made here is that collaboration in the health
system is required by environment changes; yet if it is trivial, it is
meaningless. Significant collaboration is paradigmatic, which is why
it has proved to be both difficult and poorly handled. As St. Thomas
More once said:

> It was a major provision of God's wisdom that he instituted all things on a
> community basis. Christ in his turn was highly provident when he
> endeavored to restore the spirit of community after mankind had set up
> private ownership. He saw all too well that, given the corruption of his
> nature, man's undue love of his private interests never fails to harm the
> common good.[5]

In feudal England in the Middle Ages, each village had a common
grazing ground. On this land each man put his cattle. Each added
more. Eventually there were many cattle, and each man felt that
"well, if I add only one, that won't make any difference." But
because so many villagers added cattle, the commons became
overgrazed and died. The reason the system failed was that there was

no mechanism for the villagers to understand the effects of their individual actions on everyone else, or to constrain them. This phenomenon is even more true and prevalent today, although we are perhaps also more aware that our individual actions, in our self-interest, affect conclusively, implacably, and possibly irreversibly what is available to others, which therefore ultimately affects their lives. The conflicts exist everywhere, not only in health but also in public broadcasting, in education, and even in industry. Yet we still find it hard to do much about it.

Why is this so much more of a problem today? For individuals or groups or organizations, there is now a different kind of environment from that which existed even recently, what has technically been called a state of "turbulent fields." These are rapidly changing and very complex environments in which an action of anyone in the environment affects that person and everyone else. When society was simpler, a single person, a single doctor, or a single hospital could function and make decisions as though no one else existed, and for the purposes of those decisions, that was true. Now so much changes so fast that even in industry such an attitude is untenable. A multinational manufacturing firm is so affected by changes in the value of the dollar, the cost of energy, and the cost of transporting freight that these factors may make more of a difference to success or failure than any gross efficiency or inefficiency in the way it manufactures its products.

How can one deal with such complex, rapidly changing environments? It requires reducing the uncertainty that comes from not knowing what is going to happen next and where it is going to come from, which means developing information systems that allow some degree of prediction and planning as well as having rapid decision-making processes. One group of hospitals intended to get together. As they plodded along their tortuous journey, each decision had to be passed through their separate boards of trustees. This procedure took so long that, by the time any decision had been arrived at, whatever it was that they were deciding about was no longer relevant. Thus it was twelve years before some administrator appreciated that a faster decision-making process had to be instituted. Such lags and delays are costly. In this instance, not getting together sooner cost in the neighborhood of $90 million. (Had the institutions constructed their new joint building when they first started talking, it would have cost $40 million; but when they finally built it, it cost $130 million.) Effectively dealing with change also requires influencing the environment and not simply reacting to it, in other words, being proactive. Moreover, effective influence in the face of complexity requires interdependence. Institutions just cannot go it alone anymore.

Ideally, any individual or single institution would like to be able to satisfy its designated market with its resources. But individual doctors or hospitals simply cannot do so any longer. Some hospitals, while providing excellent care in what they do do, don't have all the resources to give everything to everyone they serve. They therefore become consumers of other institutions' health care resources in the health care system. Others, like teaching hospitals, have more resources than can be effectively used in their immediate markets, so they seek out additional markets to provide for optimal utilization and essentially provide resources to the system. In the past the resource-rich, resource-poor relationships were taken care of by two means. The first was patient referral, in which hospitals with lesser resources referred patients to those with greater resources. Second, it was possible for larger health institutions to provide occasional consultation to those with need. These simple links, while still effective, are no longer sufficient. They do not deal with the problem of the complex nature of the health care system and the difficulties patients have in gaining access to what they need, when and where they need it. An integrated health care system that supplies all the necessary resources in an appropriate fashion to those that need it when they need it cannot be left to the devices of the seeker. Somehow the providers of health care resources and the consumers of them have to get together in a fashion that will enable individuals to find their way between them.

Some of the other pressures for collaboration that complicate the environment include costs that are ever escalating, gross redundancies of services, and consumers who are more demanding. Because the voluntary sector has not always spontaneously risen to the occasion, these pressures have resulted in more demanding regulation such as Public Law 93-641, which gives ten goals for planning, four of which mandate collaboration:

1. The development of multi-institutional systems for coordinating institutional health services.
2. The development of medical group practices, health maintenance organizations, and other organized systems for providing health care.
3. The development of multi-institutional arrangements for sharing support services.

4. The development by health service institutions with the capacity to provide various levels of care on a geographically integrated basis.

Almost instinctively reacting to this phenomenon, as well as to other pressures, hospitals have in fact begun to try to work together in ever increasing numbers. Soon it will be a majority rather than a minority that are at least attempting collaboration.

Some of what can be seen organizationally in the health field parallels the evolution of American business as described by Alfred Chandler.[6] Over the centuries, small businesses, as they grew larger, at first divided into yet smaller businesses before they consolidated into larger businesses that required "managing" (in the modern sense of that word) for the first time. In the early decades of this century, a further evolution took place in which many middle- to large-sized businesses consolidated through mergers. However, Chandler found that these mergers did not result in the expected increases in efficiency and effectiveness unless the businesses progressed through a further stage, namely, vertical integration. In the premerger phase, he found that businesses were still often being run by managers who were engulfed by day-to-day affairs and neglecting long-range planning.

In the health field there has been an evolution from individuals and informal groups—namely, the general practitioner or supportive neighbors—to organizations as actors in the social system such as the health maintenance organization or the group practice. This change has been in part a response to the increasing demands of and upon the health system, especially with the development of new technology that can be afforded only by relatively complex organizational structures.

FOR AND AGAINST COLLABORATION

In any health care controversy, the term "quality of care" is bandied about, especially by doctors. If a large and a small hospital talk merger, quality is immediately in jeopardy, as though poor quality were a contagious disease that might be caught. Doctors have a habit of using the term "quality of care" as something that is good and is associated with whatever it is they happen to want to do, and as something that will get lost by whatever it is anyone else wants to do that they don't want them to do. When patients express any concern with "quality of care," they think of usually getting what they want, when they want it, cheap. The community thinks of it as disposing of visible nuisances and ignoring invisible (but prevalent) ones. Let's get rid of drug addicts on the corners, but let's forget about the alcoholic in every home. Planners think of "quality of care" as anything that can be measured. Administrators define it as anything they have to do that keeps the doctors off their backs. And legislators think of it as anything that will get them reelected.

The term is nearly meaningless, or at the very least, just so much rhetoric. Consider the kind of problem that misuse of the term "quality of care" tends to create. Every hospital worth its salt has a coronary care unit. Doctors have stated that coronary care units are essential for any hospital that wishes to have high quality of care. So now each visitor to a hospital is shown with pride this small space crammed with impressive machinery. However, if one really thinks about the process of, God forbid, having a heart attack and getting treatment, then one cannot help but face the fact that most people die on the way to the hospital and that, once they are in a hospital, intervention does not make all that much difference. Once a person has physically recovered from a heart attack, the most crucial issue is whether he is going to become a cardiac invalid or not. Will he be so overcome by the possibility that any activity might be fatal that he becomes inert? Heart attack victims go through three stages: stage 1, the time elapsed between the heart attack and arriving at the hospital; stage 2, the period of acute illness; and stage 3, the recovery phase. There is considerable evidence that the existence of monitoring equipment in a cardiac care unit makes relatively little difference on the whole as to whether one survives a heart attack or not. It may be far more important to have a well-equipped ambulance that can arrive fast and give immediate attention and, equally important at the other end, to have good social and psychological rehabilitation. But neither the ambulance nor the rehabilitation are of great interest to the physician because these factors are not under his control. The cardiac care unit is, and that is where most of the money is spent.

Another argument against collaboration is that competition among hospitals is good because it keeps alert those people who might otherwise fall asleep. This very competition has led to the extraordinary redundancies and underutilization of equipment that have heavily contributed to escalating health care costs. Also, since the industry is so labor intensive, personnel expense is a major factor in driving up health care costs. Therefore, redundancy of services using people as well as machinery exacerbates the problem. Competition among hospitals within a market can no longer generally be afforded, the only exception being the unusual circumstance in which a large market exists that can support competition. It is difficult to believe that a physician would acknowledge that he would not keep on top of his profession if it were not for competition. Competition among markets, yes. Fostering competition among different hospital systems to determine who can provide the best quality of care at the lowest price would be a remarkable inducement if related to some kind of incentive.

Yet another line of reason is, "we must have it to keep our reputation." The status of an institution, its identity as a major health care entity, does not lie in its ownership of super people or marvelous things. It is use that is important, not ownership. Somehow the distinction between use and ownership must be clear cut so that it is accepted that whether doctors work at this or that institution is not as important as having them available to those in need. It is not important who owns a piece of technology; what is important is ensuring that who needs it gets served.

It should be acknowledged that there are as yet limited financial incentives to collaboration. The development of outpatient care was retarded in this country as compared with Europe because it was not reimbursed by third-party carriers until fairly recently. This situation exists today in relation to collaboration. There is relatively little incentive for institutions to do something together rather than separately as long as such new endeavors do not get some financial incentive. If they are able to achieve lower costs, then their per diem reimbursement rate is reduced, so why should they bother? Existing incentives tend to punish improvements in occupancy rates since if a rate is based on an expected occupancy of, let us say, 75 percent, and the hospital finds that it can achieve an 85 percent occupancy, then it has to return the accrued revenue and its rate will be readjusted the following year. If reducing redundancy of beds and services involves improving occupancy, which is not rewarded, no one in his right mind will do it. Pressure has to be put upon the third-party carriers to recognize and reward innovations in collaboration.

WHY COLLABORATE?
ENVIRONMENTAL IMPERATIVES

The argument for collaboration is not only financial and practical but theoretical. The environment of today, because of its complexity, requires it, as stated previously. Environments have been described as being of four types.[7] The first, called the "placid randomized environment" (type 1), is one in which goods and bads are relatively unchanging and randomly distributed. There is no distinction in organizational response between tactics and strategy. The optimal response is the simple tactic of attempting to do one's best and can be learned only on a trial-and-error basis and only for particular situations. Under these conditions, organizations can exist adaptively as single and quite small units.

More complicated is the "placid clustered environment" (type 2) in which goals and noxiants are not random but hang together in certain ways. Survival becomes precarious if an organization attempts to react to each environmental change that occurs. The emergence of strategy as distinct from tactics is important since survival becomes critically linked with what an organization knows of its environment. To pursue a goal under its nose may lead it into parts of the field fraught with danger, while avoidance of an immediately difficult issue may lead it away from potentially rewarding areas. The development of a distinctive competence, something one is particularly good at, in reaching the strategic objective is critical and requires concentration of resources. Organizations under these conditions tend to grow in size and become hierarchical with a tendency toward centralized control and coordination.

Type 3 is the "disturbed reactive environment." It is similar to types 1 and 2, but it consists of more than one organization of the same kind. Each organization has to take account of the others and also make available to others what it knows. The part of the environment to which it wishes to move may be the part to which others wish to move. So each may wish to improve its own chances by hindering the others and knows that they know this too. The organization must not only make sequential choices but also choose actions that would draw off the other organizations. It involves the development of "operations." Operations are planned series of tactical initiatives, calculated reactions, and counteractions. Flexibility encourages decentralization and puts a premium on quality and speed of decision.

The most complex environment is called "turbulent fields" (type 4). Dynamic processes that create significant changes arise from the field itself. The ground is in motion. This is a function in part of linked sets of organizations that themselves influence the environment. There is interdependence between economic and other facets of the society, and economic organizations are enmeshed in legislation and public regulation. These trends mean a big increase in uncertainty. Organizational stability under these conditions is precarious. Individual organizations, however large, cannot expect to adapt successfully simply through their own direct actions. Successful adaptation requires some emergence of new values that have significance for all members of the field as a way of dealing with the uncertainty of change and complexity. Turbulent fields demand some form of organization that is essentially different from the hierarchically structured forms to which we are accustomed. Turbulent environments require some relationship between dissimilar organizations whose fates are basically positively correlated; in other words, relationships that will maximize cooperation and that recognize that no one organization can take over the role of the other and become paramount. The executive becomes a statesman as he makes the transition from administrative management, i.e., looking after the institutions that constitute the set. Institutionalization being a prerequisite for stability, the determination of policy will necessitate not only a bias toward goals that are congruent with the organization's own character but also a selection of goals that offers maximum convergence with the interest of other parties. This series of required differences—in value, in strategy, in recognition of interdependence—amounts to a totally different paradigm in comparison with the traditional organization operating in a type 2 or 3 environment.

The development of new kinds of values includes values about the ownership of resources. A study on the Shell Refining Company shows that the company came eventually to a position where it stated that it regarded its resources, both material and human, as belonging to society as well as to itself, and it has therefore undertaken to manage these resources in accordance with this principle.[8] This particular value, a shift from absolute to conditional ownership or surrender for survival, is an apparent necessity in a type 4 environment. Those entering a type 4 environment may still continue to function in a type 3 fashion as a way of ensuring being in a good position when they get there. Thus two major hospitals in a medium-sized city, facing the possibility of having to collaborate in the near future, each built up their financial and medical resources so as to be in a better position when it came to surrendering some of their power.

Planning is critical in a type 4 environment, and the particular kind that appears to be most conducive to success is an open-ended type of planning that takes account of the emergent, allows for the unforeseeable, and follows strategies of interdependence rather than independence in resource mobilization. The strategies required to manage in this new environment are listed in the second column of the following table. Listed in the first column are those strategies that tend to characterize the health field at this time.

Existing Strategies	Strategies Required by New Environment
Responsive to crisis	Anticipative of crisis
Specific measures	Comprehensive measures
Requiring consent	Requiring participation
Damping conflict	Confronting conflict
Short planning horizon	Long planning horizon
Detailed central control	Generalized central control
Small local government units	Enlarged local government units
Standardized administration	Innovative administration

Interestingly enough, George Lodge has described the values that he sees emerging in industry and as those that industry in the near future will have to face and accept.[9] He identifies as traditional values those of individualism, property rights, competition relating to consumer desire, limited state, and scientific specialization and fragmentation. He sees as the new values, communitarianism, the rights and duties of membership, community need, active planning state, and holism interdependence. These are remarkably close to the values identified by Emery and Trist as required to operate in a turbulent environment.

The essential argument made in this book is that there are economic and social forces changing the environment in which individuals live and organizations function. The environment, as it becomes increasingly complex and unpredictable, places demands on individuals and organizations. In order to function effectively in such environments, collaboration with other organizations is required even though historically organizations have worked only for themselves, competitively or independently. This involves therefore a shift in attitude, in value, and in total world view; in other words, it requires a paradigm shift. It is because of the paradigm shift that real collaboration is, though necessary, difficult.

One further point must be added, to be reinforced below. Collaboration can be trivial or paradigmatic. Significant collaboration is essentially restricted to those structural forms in which some kind of relative irreversibility, such as merger, occurs. Intermediate forms, like consortia, promise much but are essentially unstable, for as they move to deal with important issues, they unite or, more commonly, fragment. The reason is that trivial collaboration involves unimportant, easy, or new activities. Paradigmatic collaboration implies doing differently within institutions as well as across them since the whole must be greater than the parts for collaboration to signify, i.e., there must be a reallocation of resources for improvement in efficiency, effectiveness, and integration to take place. The "trivial crisis," the confronting of "do we do as we have done before," or " do we change," occurs earlier in those structural forms that require identity melding and irreversible commitment. But it occurs in all collaborative forms affecting services (see the next chapter), and the crisis, if the structure is reversible, may precipitate withdrawal from the collaboration.

NOTES

1. Thomas S. Kuhn, *The Structure of Scientific Revolutions*, volume 2, no. 2 (Chicago: University of Chicago Press, 1970).
2. Paul R. Lawrence and Jay W. Lorsch, *Organization and Environment* (Boston: Division of Research, Graduate School of Business Administration, Harvard University, 1967).
3. R.L. Ackoff and F.E. Emery, *On Purposeful Systems* (Chicago: Aldine, 1972).
4. Irving L. Janis, *Victims of Groupthink* (Boston: Houghton Mifflin, 1972).
5. St. Thomas More, *Action and Contemplation*, R.S. Sylvester, ed. (New Haven: Yale University Press, 1972).
6. Alfred D. Chandler, Jr., *The Visible Hand* (Cambridge, Mass., and London, England: The Belknap Press of Harvard University Press, 1977).
7. F.E. Emery and E.L. Trist, "The Causal Texture of Organizational Environments," *Human Relations* 18 (1965):21-32.
8. F.E. Emery and E.L. Trist, *Towards a Social Ecology: Contextual Appreciation of the Future in the Present* (New York: Plenum Press, 1973).
9. George C. Lodge, "Managerial Implications of Ideological Change," *New York State Bar Journal*, April 1977.

Chapter 4

Types of Multi-institutional Collaboration

There are many forms of collaboration; many structural types, each with its corporate character, its legal peculiarity. This short chapter delineates the major types (see Figure 4.1). It should be appreciated that in reality pure types rarely exist. From the point of view of later chapters, the processes described therein are generally relevant, regardless of type, for the first group of forms.

Group 1, program networks, includes federation, consortium, hospital system, joint venture, consolidation, and merger. These are presented in rough order of identity retention and loss. In the former the hospitals retain identity; in the latter they lose it to some new structure or to one another. Group 2, management networks, includes shared service, hospital chain, corporation, and holding company. These are largely forms of administrative consolidation, are borrowed from industry, and their peculiarities have been well described in the industrial organizational literature. They are described here briefly for completeness and not dealt with again.

The remaining chapters present some case studies within the first group; evolutionary studies of process. The goal is to develop some sense of a generic process, later described, that may be unique to this nonindustrial group of collaborative forms. These are forms in which the collaborative purpose is not simply administrative efficiency in the traditional sense but also programmatic and service enhancement—whether efficiency or scope or integration.

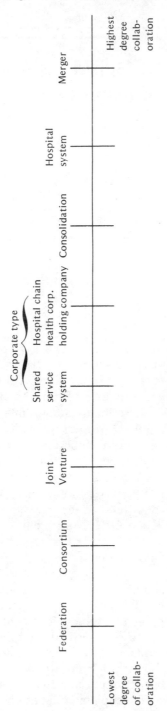

Figure 4.1. Multi-Institutional Arrangements.

GROUP 1

Federation

A *federation* is formed when several hospitals incorporate for such purposes as exchanging information, sharing services, and eliminating duplication. This is a very limited approach toward collaboration, and very informal. Cooperation is totally voluntary. Hospitals involved tend to be located within the same city or general area and draw their patients from the same population and may compete with one another or share some services. The institutions are distinct with separate identities and physical facilities. Each institution retains its separate medical and administrative staffs and maintains separate budgets. Each has its own separate board of directors.

A federation corporation usually comprises a board that includes the administrator and one trustee from each institution and one public member. Meetings of the board may be irregular. Board meetings are seen as a way of getting the administrators and trustees from each hospital to know one another better and to increase each hospital's understanding of the others. There is no special federation staff. A federation does not provide for any special planning mechanisms such as a committee other than the board members. External pressures seem to be the important factor as the impetus for collaboration, particularly government regulations.

A federation has no clout. Consequently there are very few achievements to show other than providing a forum for informal discussions. By allowing representatives from each institution to get to know each other better, it can set the stage for developing a higher degree of collaboration. Whether a federation progresses to another type would probably depend to a large degree on external pressures.

Consortium

Examples of consortium case studies are the South Middlesex Hospital Association and the Capital Area Health Consortium. While still a less committed form of collaboration, this arrangement is more advanced than a federation because the member hospitals often pay dues that support in part a salaried consortium staff. Usually this staff consists of an executive director and some assistants. The member hospitals have separate identities and physical facilities. All are located within a given geographic area and draw their patients from the same population. The consortium staff may be housed in one of the member hospitals or in a separate independent facility. The location of the staff seems to depend on historical factors and can be crucial to the survival of the consortium.

Each hospital retains its separate board, medical, and administrative staffs, and its separate budget. The executive board of the consortium usually consists of trustee, medical, and administrative representation, and it may meet monthly. There are often special committees to the board including a planning committee. Hospitals form a consortium usually because, in responding to increasing government regulation (external factors), they feel that by standing together they can increase their power against outside intervention, i.e., become some kind of lobby. The major and often only advantage of a consortium is that it allows its members to get to know one another better, like the federation. It can promote nonthreatening programs among its members and provide the hospitals with shared services, depending on its strength and the commitment of its members. A consortium board has no clout other than peer pressure. However, the fact that it has a staff and its members pay dues puts it at a more advanced stage than a federation, although they may in fact be quite similar.

Joint Venture

The joint-venture arrangement is an example of an advanced stage of the early phase of collaboration. The members coordinate their joint activities through a separate corporation. The hospitals have separate physical facilities and each member has two identities, one apart from and another together with the other members. Each has its own board, administrator, and medical staffs and its separate budget. However, there is only one administrative head for each department.

The hospitals share responsibility for some services. There is a separate board that consists of medical, administrative, and trustee representatives, and the staff is often housed in one of the hospital facilities. The presidents of each of the hospital corporations and the CEO of the joint-venture corporation are in the top management positions of the joint venture. The executive vice-president of the joint-venture corporation may have a small administrative staff. Committees to the board consist of hospital representatives. While the hospitals share services and can therefore reduce duplication, they retain their individual identities.

Consolidation

When hospitals consolidate, their administrations merge (totally integrate), while the clinical services of each institution remain intact. This system works best when the hospitals are of different types and there is no overlap of clinical services, for example, adult and children's facilities. Each facility retains its separate identity and also assumes a corporate identity. The medical staffs remain separate. Each hospital retains its own board, which becomes a division of the corporate board. The hospitals are usually located within the same physical facility. The budgets for each hospital are maintained at the corporate level. Major decisions are made by a single, central administration. There is usually a planning committee that reports to the corporate board.

Hospital System

In a "hospital system," separate institutions become divisions of a larger system. This arrangement can be brought about when one hospital purchases another and/or constructs another, and the facilities remain physically distinct while their identities are lost and they assume that of the larger system. There is usually one medical staff with all the physicians having an obligation to rotate through all the divisions. There is one administration that can be housed in one of the facilities. The divisions serve a distinct patient population and offer a similar range of services. The hospitals share and refer patients among themselves. The assets of the divisions are held centrally, while the operating budgets are controlled at both the local and system levels. Ultimate decisions regarding finances, planning, and development are the responsibility of the corporate board. A separate planning committee usually reports to the board. Unlike a consolidation, there is also usually a single board rather than separate divisional boards. A system is similar to a consolidation in that there is no separate corporate staff (as in a hospital chain or holding company), but instead there is the regular corporate structure of a single institution.

Merger

A merger (for example, Newbury) represents the highest degree of collaboration. It is the total integration of two or more institutions into (usually) a new institution with a new identity, although *acquisition* (absorption of one hospital by another) is included in this category. In this form of collaboration, individual identities are totally surrendered. Separate physical facilities and medical and administrative staffs are eliminated and replaced by one facility, one medical staff, and one administration. Since this type of collaboration usually results in the elimination of jobs, it is difficult to accomplish, and in addition, it is hard for the separate institutions to relinquish their identities. This type of arrangement probably comes about only when the hospitals involved are in extreme financial difficulties and are faced with either merging or closing.

GROUP 2

Shared-service System/Management Contracting

This setup is a hospital-based, multihospital management and service system. A shared-service system provides services for and/or manages all or parts of a group of health care facilities. The hospitals retain their separate identities and separate physical facilities. The participating hospitals are independent and serve distinct communities. Each hospital retains its separate board, medical staff, and budget. To economize, the administrators of each hospital may be paid by the shared-service system and report to it. However, individual hospital boards of trustees make their own decisions.

The reason for establishing this type of arrangement may be a need on the part of individual hospitals to improve their management structures; but more often, the reason is to facilitate purchasing services at reduced cost. Clinical services are not usually involved at all.

Hospital Chain

A "chain" is either owned and/or operated by a single corporation in which centralized services are provided to the individual hospitals. Chains tend to be more common in rural regions, as they provide a way for small hospitals to obtain economies of scale. Usually participating hospitals are independent, and each hospital retains its separate identity and at the same time takes on the corporate identity. Individual medical staffs are also maintained. An administrator who reports to one of the corporate officers is assigned to each hospital, and each hospital retains a separate board. Decisions are made at both the corporate and local level, and planning is done at this level also.

Health Corporation

A group of hospitals may also join together to form a "health corporation," which is similar to a "chain." Hospitals decide to join a health corporation usually from internal pressures, such as financial difficulties, rather than external pressures. The hospitals tend to be independent from one another and are usually located in distinct communities. Corporate officers are housed in a separate facility. Each participating hospital retains its separate identity and at the same time takes on the corporate identity. Each hospital has its own medical staff, and all decisions regarding patient care are made locally. The corporation controls the hospitals' budgets. The corporation holds "reserved powers," which entitle it to ultimate authority over budget approval and program and service development. Each hospital is responsible for its own planning. Many religious orders with dispersed hospitals have turned to this arrangement to obtain the advantages of centralized management and, for example, to improve their bond ratings, which would be lower as independent hospitals.

Holding Company

A holding company owns a group of hospitals and controls their fiscal affairs, while it leaves the actual operations and day-to-day decision-making responsibilities to the individual institutions. Each hospital retains its separate facility and identity, while also assuming the corporate identity. Each hospital has a separate board and medical staff. Individual hospital budgets must be approved by the holding company. Assets and operational budgets are held jointly. A public relations department and a planning committee are maintained at the corporate level.

This type of arrangement is very similar to a hospital chain and a health corporation except that the participating hospitals have a more established relationship among themselves and often share services and serve parts of the same communities.

Figure 4.1 outlines the various multi-institutional arrangements, on a continuum from lowest to highest degree of collaboration.

OVERVIEW OF FORMS

Geography

Program networks, the first group, are evidently limited by geography since the hospital members have to be physically adjacent to provide integrated services. Management networks are not as limited by geography. But as always, there are no pure types and many exceptions. In the shared-service system, the hospital chain, and the health corporation, all the member health care facilities are widely dispersed from one another. Each facility maintains its separate location. They serve rural communities and are similar in terms of size and clinical services available. They do not share services or relate directly to one another. The only thing they share is that they are owned and/or managed by the same corporate organization, which is physically located away from any of the individual hospitals. In the holding company, participating hospitals maintain their separate facilities but may be located relatively close together. The federation and consortium are similar types in that the group of participating institutions are situated close to one another and draw patients from the same area. In fact, the federation could be looked upon as the first step in developing a consortium. Each participating facility retains its separate location; however, the staffs of each hospital are usually familiar with one another. Because the member hospitals are usually located in or around the same city, they share common problems and pressures, which is usually the impetus for a collaboration.

In a joint venture, consolidation, or merger, the participating institutions move their original locations closer together (within the same or connected building). Patients are located in one central area, and facilities and services are combined. Because of the closer physical arrangement among the parts, there is an increase in the sharing of services and a great reduction in redundant services and facilities.

A hospital system is peculiar in that it resembles a consortium in its physical layout; however, it resembles a merger in its corporate structure. In a hospital system the parts are separate. Some of the parts have more facilities and services than others, and consequently there exists a formal referral pattern for sharing of services.

Identity

The merger and the hospital system are the only two arrangements in which the participating institutions relinquish their separate identities and assume the identity of the new organization. In the federation and consortium the participating institutions maintain their individual identities, but at the same time they take on the larger identity of the corporate organization.

It is obvious that the paradigmatic shift, in which true collaboration is confronted—that is, real efficiencies come not from new activity but only from the rethinking and redoing of old activity— occurs earlier in those forms requiring identity melding since this process is largely irreversible. Corporate structures tend not to face the trivial crisis, as collaboration is usually restricted to administrative activities and identity is not threatened.

Organizational Structure

In the merger and hospital system there is one central administration, one board of trustees, and one medical staff. All assets and operating expenses are held centrally. Decisions regarding patient care, daily operations, and special problems are made in a manner similar to that of any one institution. In both arrangements, the new organization runs as if it were one entity. There are no longer two of anything. These two types of arrangements are also similar in that the board members are responsible for scanning and spanning the environment. Each type has a planning committee responsible to the board. Decisions are usually made by consensus.

A consolidation is similar to a merger except that each institution is considered to be a division. There is one board of trustees with two divisions, and there are two medical staffs. Because a consolidation comprises two or more different types of institutions, there are often redundant departments (e.g., two x-ray departments, one for pediatrics and one for adults). Everything that can be made into one is; however, to maintain the viability of each type of institution, separate services do exist. All assets and operating expenses are held centrally by the corporation. This type of arrangement is similar to the merger and hospital system in that decisions are made at the central level, and the divisions are run by the consolidation of a single administration.

In a federation and consortium, all the participating institutions maintain separate boards and separate medical staffs. All assets and operating expenses are held by each individual institution. All decisions are made locally, and each participating hospital is totally independent. Decisions are usually made without the approval of the collaborative organization. The federation does not have a separate staff. Representatives from each of the participating hospitals, including the administrator and a trustee, meet with one another infrequently. There is no planning committee or any other committee of the board. The consortium, on the other hand, often has special staffs and committees and an executive director for the central body.

In a joint venture each of the parts maintains a separate board, medical staff, and administrative staff, but each is also part of a corporate joint-venture board. Decisions are made at both the corporate and local level, and special problems are dealt with at the corporate level. The operating budgets are maintained at the local level while their combined assets are held at the corporate level.

In the shared-service system, hospital chain, health corporation, and holding-company arrangements, the corporate structures are very much alike. Each individual hospital has a separate board, separate medical staff, and separate administration. Decisions regarding daily operations are made on the local level.

In a shared-service system engaging in management contracting, the hospitals are managed through a contractual arrangement. The administrators of all the hospitals are paid by and report to the shared-service system. However, the local board of trustees can make decisions without the approval of the shared-service system. The shared-service system acts in the role of a paid consultant. The operating budget for each hospital is controlled locally, as are the capital assets. Integration of the parts takes place through quarterly meetings of the hospital administrators. However, the parts do not relate to one another and are linked only through the shared-service system.

A hospital chain is similar to a shared-service system; however, it has more control over the hospitals it owns and/or manages, and it is considered more than a mere consultant. The administrators report to the corporate officers, and the corporation takes ultimate responsibility for its hospitals. The operating budgets and the capital assets of the parts are controlled separately and by the corporation. Many services are centralized (e.g., payroll and purchasing), and all the parts are treated alike. The hospitals are divided up by regions, and a corporate officer is responsible for a particular set of hospitals.

A health corporation is similar to a hospital chain. Decisions are made at the local level; however, the "reserved powers" the corporation holds give it ultimate authority over the individual hospitals. It is very similar to a hospital chain in that it has strong control over its hospitals. The administrators and the CEOs of the hospitals are the integrative forces between the corporation and the hospitals. Formal meetings with representatives from the hospitals are held at the corporate level on a regular basis, and the capital assets and operating budgets of the hospitals are held by the corporation. An advisory board consisting of the CEOs from all the hospitals and a corporate management staff exist to assist the corporate board. In addition to the administrators and the CEOs, vice-presidents, responsible for governing a group of hospitals in a particular region, act as liaisons between the hospitals and corporate board.

A holding company is also very similar to a hospital chain. Although it controls the hospitals, it leaves the day-to-day decision-making responsibilities to the individual institutions. Participating hospitals have an established relationship among themselves: they share services and serve different communities. The capital assets are held at the corporate level, while the operating budget is controlled at the local and corporate level. The administrators of the hospitals draw up their own budgets, which a corporate committee reviews. Each hospital has the right to approve or reject a proposed budget. Integration of the parts occurs through overlapping board membership, the senior vice-presidents, and weekly meetings with the administrators of all the hospitals. Planning takes place at the corporate level by a committee that reports to the corporate board.

Advantages and Disadvantages of Each Type

The advantage of a federation is that it gives the participating institutions a chance to get to know one another better. Because of the loosely structured arrangement, there are no concrete outcomes in terms of actual achievements. However, a federation can set the stage for greater cooperation, which is an important step in allowing the hospitals to gain trust and understanding. The disadvantage of a federation is that it has no power, and if a participating institution does not really want to go any place, it does not necessarily have to.

A consortium is similar to a federation, but it is a more concrete organization with a separate consortium staff. A consortium also sets the stage for further development, and depending on the strength of the particular consortium, it can either be ineffectual, or it can really be strong and help join the hospitals together. The advantage is that it can promote a great deal of sharing among its members. The major disadvantage is that it has no legal clout; thus if the hospitals do not want to make it work or if they want to leave the consortium at any time, they have the legal right.

Joint-venture arrangements promote a greater degree of sharing among the hospitals, and fewer services are duplicated. In addition, joint ventures can be the beginnings of strong collaborative relationships among their member hospitals. The disadvantage of the joint venture is that the hospitals are still distinct with separate boards, medical staffs, and budgets. This fragmentation necessitates redundant services. Often what begins as a joint venture (cf. the account of Affiliated Hospitals in Chapter 10) moves toward something less, or more, such as a merger.

A shared-service system, a holding company, a hospital chain, and a health corporation are all possible mechanisms for saving hospitals failing financially. The disadvantage of a shared-service system is that is has no clout. While it provides administrative expertise, it does not have ultimate authority regarding the activities of its hospitals. However, the hospitals often do improve and can expand services because of the efficient manner in which they are being run.

One advantage of a hospital chain is that it gives the hospitals' membership of a larger system for volume purchasing. The major disadvantage is that because the chain has taken ultimate responsibility for the hospitals, individual hospitals lose some of their autonomy. However, this loss is compensated by the fact that some hospitals might only survive as part of a larger system.

A health corporation is very similar to a hospital chain. The primary advantage of this type of arrangement is in its management style and system, which allow the hospitals to function more efficiently. The main disadvantage is that the hospitals lose some of their autonomy because of the reserved powers the corporation holds.

Although a holding company controls and owns a group of hospitals and controls their financial affairs, it leaves the actual operations and most of the decision-making responsibilities to the individual hospitals. The major disadvantage for these individual hospitals is that they lose a little of their autonomy.

The major advantage in consolidating is that the administration of the two (or more) hospitals merge, while the often more contentious clinical services remain separate and intact. Under this arrangement all the duplicative services in the administration are merged into one. Consolidation is ideal for hospitals offering different services. It upgrades the management of the individual hospitals while allowing them in many ways to continue to function somewhat separately. The major disadvantage to the individual parts is that they lose some of their autonomy.

The main advantage of a hospital system is that separate institutions serving distinct populations are managed by a central organization that upgrades the hospitals and makes them more efficient and effective. The major disadvantage is that there is only one medical staff and more than one physical location, which makes it difficult to hold the parts together.

The advantage of a merger is that the institutions involved become part of a larger organization that has more resources to utilize than the separate entities and is therefore stronger. When hospitals merge, they lose their identities and their former structures, and the threat in this makes it difficult to get more hospitals to agree to it. Most institutions are not willing or do not necessarily feel the need to merge.

Chapter 5

Newbury Memorial Hospital and Community Medical Center

BACKGROUND

Newbury Memorial Hospital and Community Medical Center are just under two miles apart in the town of Newbury. The next nearest hospital, Crandall, is ten miles away in a neighboring town. In 1891 an order of nuns founded the county's first hospital, St. Mary's (Community Medical Center's original name) to care for the physical ills of the residents of the community. Newbury Memorial Hospital was founded a year later with a legacy left by a Newbury resident who felt that the area needed a nonsectarian hospital. Today Newbury Memorial raises a million dollars a year from wealthy individuals and prominent corporate enterprises who have taken over many of the large estates in the still attractively wooded area. Several executives from these corporations sit on the board of trustees of Newbury Memorial.

By the 1920s Newbury Memorial had 122 beds and several clinics and was quite comprehensive for its size. Situated near a railroad, it had grown rapidly but haphazardly and occupied eight buildings

All the names and places in this chapter have been fictionalized.

supplied by eleven heating plants. The board at this time considered a move to a larger and more conveniently located facility, and three of the leading families in Newbury offered their family houses to the hospital, including twenty-four acres of land. However, the majority of the board favored moving to a different site, and most of the doctors agreed.

With the help of a generous benefactor, a new 230-bed hospital was built in 1952, although a fund-raising goal of $500,000 had not been reached. The new hospital emphasized the delivery of ambulatory care. In 1962 the Cronin Wing of 200 beds was added onto the north end of the original building, nearly doubling the hospital's size. At that time a frame for a total of nine floors was also added to be filled in later. Finally, in 1973 completion of the Wakefield Wing added another 100 beds so that today there are 541 beds. Since the early seventies the occupancy rate has risen from approximately 75 percent to more than 80 percent.

The Community Medical Center is a voluntary, nonprofit, nonsectarian general hospital serving the residents of Newbury and the surrounding area. Most recently it has been guided by a board of trustees, composed of citizens representing the community, which sets the policies of the institution. Previously it was the sectarian St. Mary's Hospital. In 1916 the cornerstone was laid for the first building of the present hospital complex. Construction of the nurses' residence in 1928, the maternity building in 1931, and the six-story main building in 1959 completed the hospital's physical facilities. In the 1950s an administrator insisted that the staff doctors sign an agreement not to supply birth-control information to patients, in keeping with the hospital's religious affiliation. Furious at this intrusion into their practices, many doctors left the staff and joined Newbury Memorial.

Later on in the 1950s, another administrator, Sister Marie, was advised by some experienced colleagues not to expand on the site because of its poor potential for future expansion. While she agreed with her advisors, her superiors decided not to relocate but instead to add on to the existing building. Coincidentally, the occupancy rate started to decline. This decline was followed by progressive increases in costs and consequent cash-flow problems, which finally led to the neglect of regular maintenance. In 1970 the occupancy rate was only 73 percent. Community Medical Center in 1977 had a licensed bed capacity of 148, including 6 ICU/CCU beds and 28 approved long-term care beds.

APPROACHES

In fall 1968 Sister Joanna, the current administrator of St. Mary's, asked Edward Boyle, the administrator of Newbury Memorial, to meet with her and her board confidentially in the office of the mother superior to discuss what Newbury Memorial might do to help her hospital. Boyle was accompanied by an attorney, John Heller, a senior bank executive, the chairman of the board of Newbury Memorial, and a retired business executive who had joined Newbury Memorial as a volunteer consultant to help with its finances for six months (but ended up staying ten years).

The Newbury Memorial group ordered a careful evaluation of the St. Mary's building by architects and engineers. The conclusion was that the physical facilities were not suitable for acute care without the expenditure of one to one and a half million dollars. The roof needed extensive repairs; the nurses' residents and the boiler room were poor; and the laundry, because it was over the boiler room, was insufferably hot. There was neither the time nor the money to evaluate the wiring and plumbing, nor the extent of compliance with the various safety codes.

Boyle and the Memorial Board concluded that they could not raise the money for this project and still conduct their own building expansion program, which was to lead to the Wakefield Wing. The Memorial Board felt that they were committed to this new construction in their role as fund raisers. The board and staff had made preliminary plans and had already paid for architects. While they felt responsible for Memorial's future, which lay in developing its excellent acute-care facilities, they felt that they would be responsible for St. Mary's only if it complemented the long-range objectives of the larger hospital. John Heller recalls that he suggested to the sisters that Memorial would enlarge its own intended addition by 100 beds to accommodate St. Mary's patients if St. Mary's could wait two or three years for them to do so. He suggested also that St. Mary's continue to operate until the new Memorial facility was completed—at which time the old building could be sold to liquidate their debts—and, moreover, that Memorial would attempt to absorb selected employees.

There were some questions about a few members of St. Mary's medical staff. It appeared that a number of general practitioners on the staff who had obstetrics and surgery privileges might not qualify for those specialties at Newbury Memorial. In fact, perhaps only half a dozen people were involved, but it seemed a large issue at the time. John Heller proposed that St. Mary's grant privileges to Newbury

Memorial's doctors immediately and that Newbury Memorial accept applications from St. Mary's MDs and use the three-year delay to remedy credential deficiencies.

St. Mary's doctors not unnaturally resisted this proposal, and stories in the press reported that Newbury Memorial would not take them on. In fact, St. Mary's was not a comprehensive medical center at that time, having only one CCU and three ICU beds; and if it had been taken over by Newbury Memorial, Memorial's staff might not have sent patients there. Memorial would have had legal difficulty defending itself in a suit if a cardiac arrest were to have occurred in St. Mary's facility. This aspect of the dilemma was not dealt with openly at the time.

Sister Joanna counterproposed that Memorial take over St. Mary's within nine months and pick up all debts, including two unrecorded notes worth $1.1 million that were debts from St. Mary's to the Mother House. The mother superior felt strongly that the Mother House was obligated to cover not only the notes but one or two mortgages and the large current payables.

FAILURE

Sister Joanna and the Memorial attorney met frequently. Nothing in the situation was attractive to Memorial except the aspect of community responsibility. At that time there was a surplus of acute-care beds, and alternative uses such as mental health and alcoholism facilities and beds were poorly funded; it was not at all clear where the operating funds for these uses would come from. In spite of exchanges, proposals and counterproposals, nothing was resolved, perhaps partly because of the long somewhat competitive history underlying the present situation. Finally, to Memorial's surprise, Sister Joanna called Edward Boyle to say that St. Mary's was closing.

Sister Joanna and Boyle worked closely together on press releases emphasizing Memorial's willingness to attempt to hire St. Mary's employees, of which there were probably several hundred. Boyle feels, in retrospect, that if St. Mary's had closed, he might have been able to pick up no more than fifty, but there would not have been a major problem since nurses and technicians were in great demand and might well have been locally employed since the area was rapidly growing with many corporations moving in. However, the closing was not to be.

At the end of January 1970, the president of the board of trustees of St. Mary's Hospital announced that the hospital would close, outlining the steps that had been taken to try and avoid this outcome. John Heller of Memorial Hospital Board issued a public statement of regret and took the opportunity to point out that there would be an interim shortage of medical facilities that Memorial could remedy with its current building program.

THE COURT INTERCEDES

The physicians at St. Mary's, extremely upset about the announced closing, took the matter to court, and the judge ruled that the hospital should not be closed at that time. This, Boyle notes, was interpreted by some to mean that the hospital should remain open, but the ruling did not in fact say this. The judge appointed a trustee to determine whether the hospital should be continued and under what conditions. The trustee, Brent Wilkes, was also appointed administrator of the hospital; he was then also chief operating officer of the State Hospital Association. The order was not appealed by Newbury Memorial because it felt that closing the hospital would have created shortages, and that their own building would not be completed for another three years. There was some difference of opinion over Wilkes's decision to keep the hospital open; Boyle believes that it should have been closed. Wilkes decided it could be viable and that a million dollars should be spent to modernize it through an FHA-guaranteed loan. The judge also created a temporary community board. Wilkes made certain plant improvements to the old building and was rewarded with headlines in the Newbury *Daily Chronicle* in December praising "how Brent Wilkes saved St. Mary's." While the hospital was supposedly operating in the black, it probably was not because depreciation was not being funded and maintenance was still neglected. Newbury Memorial went ahead with its own building program but did not put up the extra beds it had planned if St. Mary's had closed.

RENEWED APPROACHES

In June 1970, Bill Hubert, chairman of the new St. Mary's Board of Trustees, asked to meet with John Heller. In spite of glowing media reports, the situation was still deteriorating. Hubert appeared at the meeting with his whole board, provoking Heller to wonder whether communications between Hubert and St. Mary's board were as smooth as desirable. Heller wrote to Boyle later in

June suggesting that he contact Brent Wilkes for a study that might facilitate resolution of St. Mary's situation in the long-term interest of all involved, especially the community. Newbury Memorial felt an obligation to restudy the situation in depth and suspend its plans for the Wakefield Wing, concluded its current commitments, and reassessed the use of Memorial's facilities, including a special study of patient needs for physicians. The result of these deliberations was a repeat of the original offer to St. Mary's. St. Mary's once again refused the offer.

In his letter to Hubert, Heller commented on the inadequacy of the ancillary services at St. Mary's, most particularly radiology and laboratories, which he estimated would cost in excess of $1 million to remedy. He believed that St. Mary's required an equally substantial amount for additional working capital and debt capital. He pointed out that Memorial itself had only recently built fifty new beds in the shelled portion of the Cronin Wing, taxing severely its own capital funds, and that they now found themselves needing to expand their own ancillary and support facilities, and thus could not afford to take on anything new. While wanting to help, he pointed out that Newbury Memorial was presently providing nearly 85 percent of the hospital services rendered to the community, and he felt that the board's responsibility necessitated avoiding any moves that might jeopardize Memorial's commitment to patient care.

FAILURE AGAIN

Nothing therefore had changed except that St. Mary's cash position was somewhat worse. Its debt was increasing, and Memorial's capacity to help was diminished by its own expansion program. The physicians had not changed their feelings and attitudes, nor apparently had anyone else. While no one felt that it made much sense to have two hospitals in the community, no one was in a position to change that situation. It is curious that it is in this context that the glowing media reports continued, resulting in the impression being given to the community that all was returning to normal at St. Mary's.

A NEW BRUSH

In January 1971 Carl Metcalf, assistant director of a major medical center, was approached by Brent Wilkes, the court-approved custodial trustee, to replace him as administrator. While at first not interested, the more Metcalf dug into the files turned over to him, the more fascinated he became, and in July 1971 Metcalf became the CEO of St. Mary's. His understanding with Wilkes from the outset was that his job was to get the two hospitals together, not to go it alone. The court-approved plan of reorganization was very specific and involved refurbishing the facilities, restructuring the medical staff and the board, and improving the quality of services so that they would be on a par with Newbury Memorial. Essentially, the objective of the plan was to rebuild the institution to a point where it would become attractive enough for Newbury Memorial to wish to merge.

One of his first steps was to get the firm of M.M. Crowley to help with developing a strategy. Since they had prepared the Newbury Memorial strategy in the late 1960s, Metcalf presumed that they would take it into account in planning for St. Mary's. But, to Metcalf's dismay, M.M. Crowley projected St. Mary's as having a growth potential of 250 beds rather than as needing to diminish in size, as Metcalf believed they should. (His view of the situation was reinforced by the knowledge that Newbury Memorial was building 100 beds to be opened in 1973.)

A new board chairman, Michael Harrington, was appointed, and together Metcalf and Harrington started a $2.5 million capital drive for a building program. Favorable press coverage continued as a result of their aggressive public relations campaign. This program painted a somewhat rosy view of St. Mary's situation, listing 160 doctors on the medical staff (most of whom were primarily at Newbury Memorial) and a dynamic radiology department—Newbury Memorial's—which was helping them out.

When Metcalf arrived, he found that there was quite a lot of animosity at the board level between St. Mary's and Newbury Memorial. Some of this conflict dated from the souring effects of the second turndown, which led some staff at St. Mary's to feel that "we will show them we can do the job." Some of the conflict came from ancient rivalries of religion, class, and size. St. Mary's was a "gem of a little hospital offering you personalized care" versus the "big, rich, impersonal hospital." Metcalf felt that the doctors exaggerated the degree to which their privileges were threatened by close affiliation with Memorial. Their attitude was, he believed, more determined by their assessment of the effect of merger on their personal economic situation. It was true that Memorial was very selective in choosing medical staff. A number of doctors, skeptical about how much Memorial had changed its basic attitudes, had kept their affiliation with St. Mary's. Metcalf felt that the Memorial Board at that time was unprepared for a radical move, while his own board was more open to trying to work out some agreement.

Metcalf discovered that administrative memo #550 was in effect at Newbury Memorial. Dating from 1965, this memo stated that any new doctors coming into the service area of Memorial could not be on the staff of more than one hospital. This inhibited the growth of good medical staff at St. Mary's and was a major problem for Metcalf. Within two months of his arrival, he told Memorial that he would go to court if they did not change that ruling, so Memorial repealed the memo in 1971. By then, however, Memorial was so far ahead with its medical staff that it was just about impossible for St. Mary's to catch up.

Metcalf discovered that St. Mary's physical facilities had continued to deteriorate. The labs were obsolete, and the newest x-ray equipment was eighteen years old. The outpatient facilities were nonconforming, and there were minimal physical therapy and rehabilitation services. The emergency room closed its doors at 7:00 p.m., and was covered by a nurse, not a doctor, forcing ambulances to take patients to Memorial. The only in-house medical services were provided by an intern on duty, which meant that there was no real round-the-clock coverage in emergencies. To relieve the attending physicians, interns took patient histories and gave physicals, and an MD was on duty during the day for two or three hours. Pathology was controlled by a chief technician, and appointments had to be made for frozen sections. Radiology was covered by the Memorial group, but they spent only three or four hours a day at St. Mary's even though the contract called for full-time coverage. Anesthesia was administered by uncertified, foreign-trained anesthesiologists. Some medical practices were questionable, but St. Mary's medical staff seemed paralyzed in dealing with them. The fifteen trustees were well intentioned but inexperienced court appointees.

Metcalf felt that he had to:

1. Ensure that administrative memo #550 remained rescinded.
2. Reorganize the medical staff under new bylaws.
3. Restructure the court-approved bylaws for the board of trustees and its committees.
4. Obtain a Certificate of Need through the State Department of Health for the building program.
5. Enlist the support of local financial agencies.
6. Construct and refurbish a new x-ray department.
7. Refurbish the lab and the physical medicine facilities, build a small ICU and new operating suite, and build an occupational health clinic.

This second building phase took 18 months and was funded by HUD through a $2.4 million, FHA-guaranteed loan into which was folded the existing debt from phase 1 and previous financing. Phase 1 had started in September 1972. In February 1973 the Health Planning Council approved a nearly $1.6 million proposed modernization plan, and phase 2 was finished by September 1975.

While Metcalf found conflicting attitudes among the trustees and doctors, from the outset he and Gary Millen, who had become administrator of Memorial upon Boyle's retirement, worked very closely, if informally. They both agreed on the need to try to bring about some kind of resolution, and their informal meetings were reinforced by a third round of formal overtures from Harrington to Heller in 1973.

Harrington reported that they were now functioning in the black and had obtained a loan that would enable them to make the necessary physical changes to the plant. He enclosed a copy of St. Mary's long-range strategy, one of the first developed by a hospital in the state. The plan announced the change of name from "St. Mary's" to "Community Medical Center," and it included a variety of goals such as a modernization program targeting an 8-percent annual growth in inpatient utilization and a 20-percent annual growth in outpatient utilization. He suggested some areas where the two institutions could work together such as integrated planning, the administration of joint services, and possibly in some joint financing. Harrington resisted any suggestion that Community Medical Center disappear or be pushed into some narrow, specialized field such as old-age care or mental health services. He was particularly interested in exploring possibilities of working together in group purchasing, shared computer services, laundry, medical staff quality control and education, and business and accounting functions. He followed up this overture with a memorandum outlining the amazing comeback of Community Medical Center in the areas of quality and cost of health care services (the lowest daily rate in the area) and the dramatic reversal of its financial operations from an operating loss in 1969 of $207,000 to gain in the first six months of 1973 of $37,000. Another memorandum in November proposed a joint hospital task force with two trustees from either hospital and the participation of both administrators. John Heller countered with a proposal that the administrators formulate plans and present them to the trustees.

CONSULTATION FAILS

Gary Millen's joining Newbury Memorial meant that now both administrators were historically impartial and both were interested in a merger. Millen proposed to Harrington and Heller that a joint committee be set up composed of people who had not previously taken a position for or against merger. They were also exploring joint administrative possibilities, although they continued to find roadblocks in both boards. It was because of this lack of progress that the joint committee idea was activated and set up in August. Memorial was represented on the committee by the chairman of a large pharmaceutical company, an attorney, and a local businessman, all of whom were members of Memorial's board of trustees. Community Medical Center was represented by a stockbroker, a lawyer who later became a judge, and Fred Manzelli, an executive of a large corporation. An explicit condition was that the administrators not serve on the joint committee. The joint committee was spurred on somewhat by the pressure Community Medical Center was now beginning to feel from the new state reimbursement system that favored hospitals with more than 200 beds. During the period of the joint committee and subsequent consultant studies, Metcalf accomplished his goals of completing the renovation of the radiology department, modernizing lab services, relocating and expanding physical therapy, and drastically overhauling the ICU and CCU. Relocation, expansion, and modernization of operating suites and existing emergency and outpatient services were also completed, and many new services were implemented.

Fred Manzelli, director of corporate affairs at a large corporation where his superior was Michael Harrington, had served on a regional health planning council, of which he became president in 1975. He joined the board of Community Medical Center in 1973, eventually succeeding Harrington as chairman in 1977.

Manzelli provides some insight into the functioning of the joint committee. It met at the Newbury Club, a venerable institution. The main mission of the first meeting seemed to be what to choose for dinner. Manzelli's own position on the committee was challenged immediately because of his membership in the regional planning council, which some members felt reflected a planning process that was increasingly asserting itself into the affairs of local hospitals. Periodic committee meetings seemed unable to focus on the issues at hand and concentrated instead on the selection of the proper consultants to examine both hospitals in the light of community need and fiscal viability. The committee decided to hire a consulting team to help determine whether each hospital should go it alone, share services, or join in some form of merger. The hospitals were to share the cost of the study proportionately according to the number of beds in each.

Manzelli remembers that the consulting team lost credibility, as they tended to argue among themselves in front of their clients.

Their first tentative report at the end of 1975 suggested, much to everyone's surprise, that Community Medical Center could indeed go it alone.

Metcalf resigned in January 1976 and was replaced temporarily by Harold Miller, a vice-president in the State Hospital Association. Metcalf left having accomplished his original goals of improving the physical facilities and services but at the great price of incurring a debt of $2.4 million. He had accomplished much, including establishing a working relationship with Gary Millen at Memorial. But in spite of Metcalf's efforts within the hospital, the new state reimbursement system did not favor small institutions with less than 200 beds, and the impact and effects of this system started to become clear about three years after its initiation, just when Metcalf was preparing to leave. So in early 1976, Community Medical Center, with better plant and facilities and some increase in patient days, was in a more desperate operating financial position than ever. The Department of Health required the hospital to reduce operating expenses by $612,000, to terminate thirty-five full-time positions, and to place a wage freeze on all remaining personnel if it was to operate within its approved per diem rate for Blue Cross and Medicaid patients. Debt service on the loan plus minimal increase in patient utilization left the operating cash position equally poor. In spite of the improvements in physical plant, the increased debt made Community Medical Center even less attractive to Newbury Memorial.

One Memorial representative on the committee responded sharply to the consulting team's initial report, which suggested that Community Medical Center was viable. He was not impressed at the apparent surplus Community Medical Center reported for the previous three months and recognized that merger still meant assumption of Community Medical Center indebtedness. He was also aware that the state was losing patience with Community Medical Center as a high-cost operation and wondered aloud whether the consultants were correct. He felt that if the consultants were correct, there might be some advantages to merger, but that if they were wrong, it might be disastrous; therefore he suggested great caution.

His apprehensions were confirmed by a phone call from the consultants to another Memorial representative a few days later, in which the consultants corrected some of their earlier conclusions and stated that Community Medical Center not only would not be able to make it on its own as an acute-care facility but would be out of business in one to three years. The team's conclusions that the only possible salvation for Community Medical Center would be full merger with Memorial were presented on April 8, 1976, to the joint planning committee of the two boards. The team proposed proceeding with an analysis of the financial implications of full merger, but the committee wanted time for consideration before spending more money on surveys.

The committee was deeply concerned about a further extension of the study by the consultants in view of their total turnabout in their prediction of the future of Community Medical Center. The medical director of Memorial, irritated at the wasted planning time resulting from the consultants' change of heart, proposed, not for the first time, that all acute care should be consolidated at Memorial and that Community Medical Center, even if merged with Memorial, should be used for ancillary purposes such as extended care or psychiatry. Other criticism of the interim consultant report was directed at the fact that the consultants had not been hired to propose merger but to evaluate alternatives. On April 23, 1976, the joint committee expressed its dissatisfaction directly by terminating the study.

The consultant report did help to educate the trustees at Community Medical Center, and forced them, as Fred Manzelli said, to take a harder look at themselves. He had by now succeeded Harrington as chairman of the Community Medical Center Board, and his understanding of the planners and planning helped him in his new role. His quite different orientation facilitated an attitude change among doctors and trustees that was eventually to lead to a breakthrough in the deadlock.

Later that year Community Medical Center's board authorized its independent auditors to conduct a special study and analysis of fiscal operations as a follow-up to the terminated consultant study to clarify which, if any, of the study results were correct. Community Medical Center continued cost reductions and cutbacks where it could. The auditor's report was a not unanticipated shock to the Community Medical Center Board. It not only confirmed the consulting team's gloomy predictions but said matters were even worse than when the consultant study was done. Community Medical Center was losing half a million dollars a year, not just because of the reimbursement system but because of management problems. The emergency room was losing $130,000 a year; the executive health program, which should have been profitable, was also in the red; the day-care program was costing $60,000 a year; and the medical staff was not supporting the hospital with increased admissions.

In October 1976 Fred Manzelli and Harold Miller of Community Medical Center met with Gary Millen of Memorial and concluded that the auditor's substantiation of the consultant study meant that Community Medical Center had no alternative but to work out something with Memorial or declare bankruptcy. They felt that it was time that the administrators be included in the joint committee membership, and a question was raised as to whether Memorial might provide administrative services to Community Medical Center while any subsequent studies were being made. Such studies, they felt, should focus on specialized uses of the Community Medical Center facilities, a move not previously favored by Community Medical Center trustees and doctors. A newspaper article in early November 1976 reflected for the first time Community Medical Center gloom and publicized the question of conversion or merger. Involvement by Memorial in a management contract with Community Medical Center was vetoed by Memorial's counsel in view of the potential damages that could be incurred if Community Medical Center went bankrupt and claims were made that it was acting on the part of Memorial.

The vice-president for planning at Memorial prepared a brief for John Heller in which he concluded that Community Medical Center as presently constituted was not viable and that there was no need for the acute-care facilities that it represented. He recommended some alternative short- and long-term uses that might have value for Memorial if conversion could be carried out.

A MANAGEMENT FIRM
COMES AND GOES

1977 was an eventful year. In the spring the deputy commissioner of the State Department of Health expressed the view that there was no future for Community Medical Center as an acute-care facility. Negotiations continued with Memorial. In May, Alan Hadley, executive director of the local Health Systems Agency, proposed that the joint planning committee include the administrators and work with the HSA to find a solution. The idea of outside management running Community Medical Center that was proposed in late 1976 now became a reality. An outside management firm was retained on July 11 to manage Community Medical Center, but the year ended with the firm in disarray. In December a crucial meeting between Community Medical Center, Memorial, and the Department of Health took place.

In early January 1977, Memorial's attorney wrote to Fred Manzelli reporting the results of the November joint committee meeting.

Memorial reiterated its position that it could not assume Community Medical Center liabilities and that any of the community's acute-care needs would better be taken care of by expanding Memorial. Memorial's position continued to be that Community Medical Center should explore with the State Department of Health and the HSA its possible uses to the community for some form of ancillary and extended care.

Memorial's view was backed by a letter from the Department of Health's deputy commissioner, who said that he was impatient with what was essentially a public subsidy of Community Medical Center. Manzelli found the letter disturbing and said so. The deputy commissioner therefore suggested that the hospital and the department meet together with representatives of the HSA.

Manzelli called a meeting of representatives from Community Medical Center and Memorial in mid-March and restated his view that Community Medical Center could continue in the acute-care business for the foreseeable future. However, he also announced that the board would look for the first time at alternative uses for its facilities. He then mentioned that they were negotiating with an outside management company. Each hospital supported the desirability of keeping one another informed as to plans and programs, but it was not clear to the Memorial representatives why Manzelli had called the meeting in view of the generalities discussed.

The initiative the deputy commissioner suggested was taken up in May by Alan Hadley, who invited both hospitals to reconvene the joint committee and meet with the HSA. John Heller responded that the joint committee was awaiting any further proposals by Community Medical Center and that if Hadley had anything concrete to suggest, it would be more appropriate for him to meet with Heller, Manzelli, and the two administrators rather than with the joint committee.

With the employment of the outside management firm for Community Medical Center, consolidation of the services of the two hospitals appeared dead for the time being. Mark Wittenberg was appointed administrator of Community Medical Center for the outside management firm as part of a three-year contract. In mid-November, Wittenberg reported to Manzelli a series of recommendations and alternative courses of action resulting from four months of analysis. Overwhelming problems having been identified in the business office and accounting department, it was the management firm's considered opinion that the Community Medical Center operation as an acute-care facility should terminate no later than

December 31, 1977. The firm based its conclusion upon: accounts payable of $1.3 million, a grossly insufficient cash surplus; the likelihood of large deficit in 1978 on the basis of an average daily census of fewer than eighty-eight patients; and a reimbursement rate that, while possibly satisfactory for 1978, would certainly be pushed down by the Department of Health in subsequent years once the subsidy to the calculated rate of reimbursement was discontinued. The pension plan was illegally underfunded, and physician support was eroding. While some money might be realizable by selling off property, not enough could be raised by this method to solve the essential problem.

Wittenberg proposed that Memorial acquire Community Medical Center and convert it to an extended care facility or detoxification center. He also suggested the alternatives of bankruptcy or selling Community Medical Center privately as a nursing home.

Manzelli arranged a meeting quickly with the Department of Health in mid-November of 1977 after receipt of the management firm's report. The deputy commissioner was relieved that the Community Medical Center Board, with or without the concurrence of its medical staff, had decided that it could not make it on its own. He telephoned Millen at Memorial to ask him to arrange a meeting between the commissioner of health and his staff and the leadership of both hospitals to explore what could be done on behalf of the community. He pledged the department's full support to solve a problem that plagued the Department of Health, the community, and *both* hospitals. (This is perhaps the first time that everyone acknowledged being part of the problem.) The meeting was arranged for December 6, 1977.

A flood of newspaper stories reported on the meeting in December of the state health commissioner with representatives of Memorial and Community Medical Center. He was accompanied by the deputy commissioner and a representative from the Health Care Facilities Financing Authority. The commissioner favored Memorial's acquisition of Community Medical Center, the indebtedness of which was estimated to be $3.8 million. His proposal was that Memorial assume Community Medical Center's debts by floating thirty-year bonds at 7-percent interest, a move that would add approximately $2.00 to Memorial's per diem rate. The press did not hesitate to point out that the Regional Health Planning Council had recommended seven years previously that Community Medical Center be closed when St. Mary's wished to terminate operations. The press also brought the name of Crandall Hospital into the picture for the first time as a possible partner with Memorial in any takeover of

Community Medical Center for use in their contemplated jointly operated (consortium) Center for Addictive Illnesses.

Newspaper reports noted Memorial's foot dragging, with some papers criticizing what they saw as parochialism and even lack of concern for the provision of adequate health care in the community. The press stories led John Heller to write the newspapers an open letter in which he reminded the public that the board of trustees of Newbury Memorial had always affirmed the primary mission of that hospital as providing acute medical care and that Memorial should not divert its resources from its primary mission. But he added that if a need were identified by the Health Systems Agency, then Newbury Memorial would work alone or in cooperation with others to serve that need on a responsible and economically viable basis. In other words, he put the ball clearly in the HSA's court.

There were some interesting dynamics underlying the December meeting that were not perhaps totally apparent to those who read the newspapers. On the face of it, the commissioner's proposal was a possible way for Memorial to assume increased debt; however, it would have cost the community many millions more than the existing outstanding debt at the proposed rate of 7 percent annually for thirty years. The commissioner was highly motivated to resolve the situation since the newly reelected governor had not reappointed him as a member of his cabinet. It was felt by some that if a hospital such as Community Medical Center went bankrupt under the system designed by his administration, his reappointment might be in question. He became frustrated in the meeting when Memorial did not readily agree to his proposal. Memorial, on the other hand, had anticipated a proposal it could study, while the commissioner was intent on having a letter of agreement in principle before the first meeting adjourned. Behind Memorial's hesitation was the conservative attitude of its trustees who were traditionally concerned with preserving Memorial's solvency.

The meeting ended dramatically when the deputy commissioner received a telephone call. In the middle of the deadlocked negotiations, he reported that they had found another hospital that might be interested in taking Community Medical Center over if Memorial had no objections. Memorial was then asked to leave the room while the commissioner's staff talked and was not told the identity of the mystery suitor. Hadley of the HSA was present at the meeting, and he pointed out that Community Medical Center could not negotiate with anyone unless the HSA had assessed community needs, and no one had yet requested such an assessment.

BANKRUPTCY AND MERGER

When Gary Millen first arrived at Memorial, it was traditional for the 133 trustees to meet three times a year to review reports on the hospital's condition and to ratify the proposals of the 28-member executive committee. This committee met monthly to receive reports of the active committees. While it can be said that the board of trustees was totally committed to the hospital, the infrequent meetings of the body as a whole made their education on health issues difficult. It was difficult to call more frequent meetings mostly because of the board members' commuting and the other community activities in which they were involved. Yet it was to this group that the administration looked for guidance.

Millery had recommended the establishment of a bylaws committee to review the board structure and to recommend changes that would be appropriate to the present climate in which trustee education would be more feasible, the decision-making process could be expedited, and the liability of the 133-member board could be reduced if it could not be persuaded to meet longer and more frequently. The bylaws committee of 6 included two chairmen from two prominent corporations, an attorney, two other corporate executives, and the head of a women's association. The committee proposed and set up a membership corporation with no other legal responsibility or authority than to elect trustees. The new chairman desired more local input in the composition of the new board. The new board of trustees was to consist of the hospital administrator, the medical director, the president of the medical staff, the chairman and vice-chairman, and 20 others. On November 1, 1977, this major revision to the bylaws was instituted, and the new board took office in February 1978. The new board immediately identified the Community Medical Center situation as one of Memorial's major community responsibilities. The board said it would weigh action after receipt of Part II of the HSA report and comments from the HSA public hearing that was ultimately held on April 5, 1978.

On January 1, 1978, the HSA had produced Part I of two reports with the conclusion that no additional acute-care beds beyond those supplied by Memorial were needed in the Newbury area. The HSA did point out that if there were no other acute-care facilities in Newbury, Memorial would have to operate at a maximum efficiency and reduce patient stay through the use of preadmission testing, outpatient surgery, increased home health agency referrals, and the developing health maintenance organization in the county.

On January 26, 1978, the board of trustees of Community

Medical Center announced that the hospital would be placed in receivership under Chapter 11 of the Federal Bankruptcy Act, and so informed its medical staff. The Community board felt that this action would buy time in which to develop and present a positive case for the reorganization and continuation of the hospital as an acute-care facility. The action also was intended to keep the creditors at bay, a major one being the outside management firm. Part of the crisis had been produced by the state's withdrawal of its rate subsidy so that Community Medical Center's cost of $155 a day was reimbursed by only $133. The action, under the reorganization statute, meant that creditors who might have taken Community Medical Center to court to seize its assets were put off at least for a while. Even at this point, the Community Medical Center medical staff, headed by Dr. James Ditolla, was still pushing for the continuation of acute-care services, and it was their adamant position that, while initially supported by their trustees, eventually led to the ultimate resolution of the problem. The president of the Memorial medical staff wrote to Dr. Ditolla expressing his sympathy and, in the event of Community Medical Center's ceasing to provide acute care, offering to expedite integration of the medical and dental staffs.

Later in the month of February, a retired state supreme court justice was named receiver by the bankruptcy court. (Remarkably, in the light of these events, Community Medical Center was reported in one local paper to be having record-high patient admissions! The Community Medical Center physicians who had hired a public relations firm to carry their campaign to the public were clearly getting good mileage for their money.)

The outside management firm resigned from its contract effective February 28, 1978, with $140,000 unpaid on its contract. The doctors' public relations program rolled relentlessly on, and in late February a poll reported that the public wanted Community Medical Center to stay open as a full-service hospital. In spite of this, Part II of the HSA plan was released, which noted that the local community's consumer views still remained to be solicited. The plan proposed three alternatives for Community Medical Center as first-priority considerations:

    a. A multiservice regional outpatient and inpatient psychiatric facility.

    b. A regional center for alcoholism treatment.

    c. A comprehensive-care center for the developmentally disabled.

There were other possibilities, but the three just listed corresponded to what the HSA identified as the needs of the community. A second priority would be the development of health services for the aged such as a long-term care facility specializing in posthospitalization extended care or a sheltered-care facility. This report, released in late February, produced a flood of media coverage during March and April, much of which appeared to be a carefully orchestrated outpouring of support for Community Medical Center to continue as an acute-care facility. Dr. Ditolla sent the HSA a compromise proposal of 80 medical/surgical beds (down from the licensed 120) with an additional 30 being devoted to short-term psychiatric care. He proposed also continuing Community Medical Center's 26-bed extended-care unit. Hospital audits at this time reported that its financial position was not apparently quite as bad as had been suggested and that it could remain in operation at least through the end of April.

News stories reported all kinds of suggestions for new roles for Community Medical Center, some of which derived from the HSA's proposals, and a key one being the creation of a Center for Addictive Illnesses (CAI) to be operated jointly by Crandall and Memorial, already consortium partners who were developing a Certificate of Need for a freestanding CAI.

The HSA held a public hearing on April 5, which it asked the county advisory council to host, but the chairman of that council raised a question as to whether the HSA should be involved because the facility was in receivership. Hadley's sharp reply was that the HSA had been involved repeatedly with the parties concerned and with the state health commissioner, and he had fully informed the court-approved receiver of the HSA role in the negotiations. He reminded the chairman of the council that, eight years before, the Community Medical Center trustees had spent several million dollars upgrading a hospital that was now bankrupt, seemingly a justification for regional planning involvement. Nevertheless, the advisory council did not choose to be present, and the meeting was conducted by the HSA. At this meeting an emotional outpouring of public affection for Community Medical Center was expressed by nurses, doctors, employees, and ex-patients. But the die was cast.

Bob Dickinson had by now been appointed the new administrator by the receiver and was able to achieve some useful short-term financial results. At this point in time Manzelli felt that all the trustees at Community Medical Center were now clearly in favor of merger, and many of the doctors had swung in this direction with only a few hard-liners remaining. Clearly the hospital's closing was a political issue, because 300 lost jobs in a community of that size would make headlines. Since the State Department of Health had several hospitals in Community Medical Center's situation and had been directly involved for some time, it was particularly interested in using the case as a model for solving the problem of closing a small hospital while preserving jobs, a big issue in the state.

St. John's a hospital located about ten miles away, at this time expressed interest in Community Medical Center, and Community Medical Center was in touch with them as a possible partner while continuing to explore possibilities with Memorial. Fred Manzelli felt that his job at this point was to orchestrate and mediate. He was not sure whether this role also involved using St. John's as a stalking horse. It should be noted that the mysterious suitor of the commissioner's December 6 meeting was Crandall Hospital, Memorial's consortium partner. Crandall had been ignorant of the developments at the commissioner's meeting, and when a member of the health department asked if they would look at Community Medical Center as a possible CAI, they innocently replied affirmatively.

In mid-April Gary Millen met with Fred Manzelli and Dr. Ditolla, as well as the new chairman of the Memorial Board. Manzelli and Ditolla wanted Memorial's impressions of the compromise physicians' plan. Millen told Manzelli that he had received authorization from his board at their April 5 meeting (the evening of the HSA afternoon public hearing) for a feasibility study on acquiring Community Medical Center. The following week he met with Memorial's accountants, and he continued to hold frequent meetings with them over the next weeks. Ten days later a subcommittee of the board, chaired by the president of a major insurance company's regional operations, met with Millen, the accountants, the deputy commissioner from the Department of Health, and the director of the state bonding agency. The purpose of the meeting was to get the deputy commissioner's support for the financial arrangements necessary. The deputy commissioner proposed a single reimbursement rate for both hospitals and funding short-term debt of $1.3 million, and long-term debt of $2.7 million by bond issue or as an add-on to the reimbursement. He felt that Certificate of Need questions could quickly be resolved.

The newspapers duly reported these negotiations and the proposal to use Community Medical Center as a "Center for Addictive Illnesses." Memorial, however, commented only that its use of the facility was to be consistent with the HSA recommendations and that its primary concern was to preserve the jobs of the employees and the assets of Community Medical Center for the health needs of the community. Media stories still appeared supporting Community

Medical Center's continuation in acute care and in this context introduced St. John's as being prepared to support the Community Medical Center physicians' plan of two-thirds acute care and one-third psychiatric beds.

During May the Newbury Memorial Board and administrators continued drawing up a plan with the help of their accounting firm and with input from appraisers, architects, engineers, and pension consultants. The accountant's interim report was agreed to by the Memorial staff on May 5, 1978. Three days later the board's subcommittee met with the Community Medical Center medical staff's leadership and continued to meet over the next several days. The Community Medical Center physicians' position was not helped by a report released by Bob Dickinson to the medical staff on May 10 noting extensive medical chart delinquencies amounting to almost 50 percent of an entire year's discharges and representing a serious licensing deficiency. Under the previous suspension system, forty-nine physicians would have been suspended, but Dickinson, with the agreement of the court-appointed receiver, did nothing because the result would have lowered admissions and further reduced the hospital's ability to remain open. This information, however, was probably instrumental in undercutting the last vestiges of resistance to any reasonable plan that Memorial might put forward.

On August 15, 1978, Community Medical Center officially became part of Newbury Memorial Hospital. The plan involved phasing out acute care and introducing skilled nursing beds and ambulatory care over the succeeding twelve months. A Certificate of Need would be requested for the immediate conversion of forty acute-care beds to long-term care, and the Center for Addictive Illnesses proposal would be pursued as well as a program for rehabilitation medicine. The court-appointed receiver had the last word: He said the merger was "frankly, something I didn't think we'd be able to do."

Chapter 6

Cancer Collaboration Association

In September 1973 there was a conference on cancer control sponsored by the National Cancer Institute in Columbia, Maryland to promote interest in model cancer management systems. Subsequently a number of cancer centers were encouraged to submit applications to the National Cancer Institute for development grants, and several of these were funded in summer 1974. One such funded center was the Cancer Control Center (CCC). The CCC was invited to work with a major cancer hospital, one of four hospitals in a Midwestern town, but counter proposed a consortium in the town as a model cancer management system, involving all four institutions. The hospitals were skeptical, as competition among them had received considerable attention within the community and communication among the administrators was strained. The goals of the CCC application were to develop a collaborative working arrangement around sharing resources and sharing expertise by, for example, making oncologists available to other hospitals. CCC and the hospitals were able to negotiate a collaborative arrangement that was limited to the four hospitals but involved developing outreach programs through the increased use of social work, community agency involvement, and nursing. There were, even prior to the consortium, many multiple appointments of physicians and referrals among the hospitals.

At approximately the same time as these negotiations were being held, the State Department of Public Health was proposing to establish standards for cancer management in an effort to upgrade the quality of cancer care. The Department of Public Health's efforts followed the National Cancer Act of 1971, which specifically called for the director of the National Cancer Institute to "establish programs as necessary for cooperation with state and other health agencies in the diagnosis, prevention and treatment of cancer." It is therefore not surprising that the actions of the Department of Public Health made hospitals, and especially physicians, extremely apprehensive, as it now seemed clear that they were going to be told whom to treat and how to treat them.

Coincidentally, the Cancer Commission of the American College of Surgeons, under a subcontract for the Cancer Advisory Committee, had made some assertions about the management of cancer; namely, that a cohesive regional stratified system of care should be developed that would link institutions with limited resources to those of more complete resources; that hospitals be encouraged to develop plans for care that would avoid unnecessary duplication; that care should be provided as close to home as possible, taking into account the medical, financial, and psychological implications for the patient; and that channels for consultation, referral outreach, and continuing education be established. These assertions implied the designation of those hospitals that provided care for cancer patients into three broad categories of hospitals plus a fourth category devoted to the treatment of special cancers of special groups of patients. The categorization consisted of: (category 1) hospitals providing comprehensive specialized services and advanced specialty training and research; (category 2) hospitals providing comprehensive specialized services; and (category 3) hospitals providing basic and selected services; or (category S) hospitals providing basic services primarily in hospitals providing services for special types of cancer or special groups of patients.

The Cancer Advisory Committee's assertions had a number of operational and substantive implications for the hospitals, particularly for those doing work categorized for types 1 and 2 institutions yet having those resources classified as type 3.

Therefore it was not surprising that a reason frequently given for the subsequent development of what became the Cancer Collaboration Association (CCA) was that it was a defensive move against the impending development of the Health Systems Agency (HSA). The hospitals felt that the HSA was likely to impose plans on them and that to preempt this they should get together and form their own planning group that could influence and head off unwanted acts on the part of the HSA. The CCA was clearly a beginning toward such a group, and in the discussions of the CCA's future, many believed that it should move toward some kind of general association or hospital consortium.

With this background in mind, it becomes easier to understand the ambivalence that existed on the part of CCA institutions about becoming actively involved in a collaborative venture of any sort that would limit their autonomy or prescribe new behavior modalities. It also becomes easier to understand the significant challenge that the CCC faced when it negotiated a collaborative arrangement among the four hospitals, recruited a local staff, and set up an organization.

The CCA staff were three in number—nurse, administrator, and physician—and each had been selected with the approval of their appropriate constituency in the hospitals. The site of their office, chosen with care and forethought and placed in a downtown office building, represented a neutral place away from the four member institutions. While they worked closely with the CCC, they obtained their primary direction from the CCA board and regarded themselves as staff to it.

An eleven-member board was created consisting of three members (physician, administrator, and trustee) from each hospital, a community representative, and a staff member of CCC who stayed on as a neutral chairman at the hospitals' request. Each board member had one vote. Committees were created in the areas of research and funding, data and information, care and treatment, cooperative cancer education, and oncology nursing. These committees were chaired by CCA staff and consisted of nonboard representatives from the hospitals. A range of activities were started.

After about a year of activity, much of it organizational in nature and apparently quite unpublicized, in the winter of 1975 the board voted to invite the five remaining acute-care hospitals in the rural area surrounding the town to join CCA.

Initially the CCA offered the five rural hospitals only one vote each on the board, in contrast to the original four urban hospitals, because the CCA believed that the board could not mandate its role as an executive committee if it were to increase so drastically in size. Also the urban four did not wish to be outvoted by the rural five, especially since the latter were perceived as less sophisticated providers of cancer care. However, the rural five obtained three votes each.

ACTIVITIES

The CCA's many activities had generally been initiated by the board, by the committees, or most often by CCA staff. There appeared to be no special rationale for them, although an early strategy was to improve institutional relationships and reduce defensiveness by avoiding controversial activities. Certainly, the staff's intention was to facilitate the hospitals' working together. Activities proposed by the staff were discussed and approved by the committees and board. The major activities are reviewed below:

1. *The Central Tumor Registry:* All member institutions seemed to be at least superficially interested in the establishment of a central tumor registry. Yet there appeared to be a considerable disagreement about the purposes of establishing such a registry as well as about duplication. Should the various hospitals that at the time had one, keep their own? Would a loss of autonomy occur if all data was fed into a central registry and lost to the individual institutions? It seemed clear that the central registry would be useful, especially in the long run to health planners and to administrators who were making capacity decisions, although it was not clear how physicians would use the data in a way that would influence the kind of care they give. It was also not clear whether individual hospitals were willing to pay for the use of the registry.

2. *Education:* All the institutions appeared to be interested, although to varying degrees, in the educational efforts that CCA had coordinated. The various institutions did not have to commit themselves financially to any of the educational programs and could benefit from them without committing the time of their physicians or administrators. Education was seen as the major gain as a result of CCA, yet while the purpose of this activity had been to foster interhospital communication, meetings at a specific institution had been far better attended by the host hospital staff than by others. The reasons for this attendance pattern seemed to be that it was difficult to leave one's patients and intrahospital activities even for a short period of time, particularly when the scheduled meeting was across town. Also, since it had not been given priority, increased participation, especially on the part of physicians, had simply not occurred. Educational efforts aimed at nurses were more successful, at least if one assumes that success is measured by attendance. Yet because a number of these meetings had been

developed in conjunction with the American Cancer Society, it was once again difficult to sort out the impact of CCA.

3. *The Development of Standards:* A major activity since the inception of CCA had been to develop screening forms to be used by physicians at participating institutions in order to standardize the management of a particular disease. To date, the activity had centered mostly on breast cancer, and the utilization of these forms varied widely. The sanctions for not using the forms also varied. While a number of institutions felt that utilization was and should remain completely voluntary, others planned to make the form a part of patient history procedures and thus censure any physician who did not completely fill out the forms.

CCC AND CCA STAFF

The CCC's assumptions were based on a tradition of helping local communities and health agencies upgrade their own facilities. It had certain expectations about acting as a resource, as a training facility, and as a consultant in diagnosis and treatment. The CCC saw its role not in providing programs for local communities but in helping them obtain the benefit of a wider range of resources. The CCC's assumptions were:

1. The capacity of the community hospital to provide optimal care could be increased by pooling resources among as many professionals as possible.
2. The services provided by community hospitals and community professionals were the central strengths of the medical care system.
3. The quality and outcome of cancer care could be improved by modifying the existing health delivery system.
4. Optimal care should be provided as close to the local community as possible.
5. Formal arrangements among institutions were necessary to include the services of specialists in cancer care.

The CCC's goals were to encourage interhospital cooperation and community-wide linkages; to encourage the hospitals to use certain standards for screening; to develop guidelines for the management of cancer care; to develop guidelines for audit; and to transfer "state-of-the-art" capabilities to physicians through professional education programs to change physician behavior.

The board chairman felt that it was nearing the time to hand over more of the leadership to the local institutions.

The three members of CCA staff worked individually with their respective constituencies—physician with the physicians, administrator with the administrators, and nurse with the nurses.

The physician felt that the development of standards was a high priority. Thus standards were developed by a committee of physicians, which worked on the standards forms. These forms were then presented to the board, and if approved, they were submitted to each hospital's review committee, which could accept them for trial or request revision. The committee's essential objective was to develop quality-assurance documents within hospitals. In addition, the forms were intended to reduce the amount of omitted or incorrect data. The committee's approach in creating the forms was to avoid controversial areas.

The nurse focused on developing professional education programs for the hospitals and standard nursing care plans that might be used by all hospitals to obtain better nursing care. She worked closely with the regional unit of the American Cancer Society in her educational efforts, and she intended to initiate activities and then hand them over to local institutions.

The administrator was chairman of the committees on data and information, and research and funding. His goal was to obtain sources of funds through the research and funding committee and to develop a data system for CCA through the committee on data and information. He had spent a lot of his time on organization, such as the memorandum of understanding between the hospitals, and on building liaison, especially with the rural five hospitals. The five hospitals, he felt, joined only because two years before the state had threatened imposition of management regulations. He expressed some concern with the evolution of CCA as to whether it might end, become a hospital consortium beyond cancer treatment, extend to more agencies or become the quality-assurance agency for cancer treatment.

He felt that technically if the board agreed to a set of treatment guidelines, the nature of the memorandum of agreement was such that this was mandated upon the hospital nonmembers. This fact was appreciated by the urban four but not by the rural five. The trustees tended to back the administrators, but the administrators made little effort at that time to educate the trustees, except those few on the board.

THE URBAN FOUR:
PERCEPTIONS
AND VALUES

Administrators of the urban four seemed to feel that they had capabilities in oncology care, but the problem was distributing it better, especially to the periphery. They saw the CCA staff as their own rather than as autonomous professionals. One administrator said that the CCA was born under compulsion and enlarged in paranoia. He felt that it was not self-generating and only existed, like any grouping, where there was a common threat or common thread. The latter, he believed, did not exist. Eventually, he believed, the CCA had to evolve into a chain or a consortium, but at this point the enlargement represented a state of indigestion.

The main problem seemed to be the fact that dollars were available for administrative support, but not for programs and would terminate in the future. The administrators felt that there was significant need for regional programs and that support for them would not be available from the grant; thus the need as they perceived it would not be met by the present grant. They also felt that the CCA was an expensive operation, and they were concerned with the development and high cost of the central tumor registry versus local registries. They felt that the central tumor registry was not a substitute for the local registry, and quoted the American College of Surgeons as being against central tumor registries. The role of the CCA staff was unclear to them, and some felt that what was being done was not what was most needed, i.e., that priorities were wrong. Finally, attendance by hospital representatives at critical meetings was felt to be less than optimal.

Some of the hospital administrators felt that little had been accomplished except for some organizational evolution, but others felt that the CCA at least represented a catalyst with possibilities and that it had a neutral chairman with the capacity of objectively resolving or reconciling interinstitutional conflicts. The quality-of-care activities had taken most of the CCA's effort to date. The tumor conferences/boards had probably been good, while the standards forms probably had taken too much of the CCA's time. One of the CCA's accomplishments was the coordination of screening guidelines, although the extent of implementation in the hospitals was poor.

The administrators agreed that interaction among physicians had improved, as had their attitudes, and that they seemed to be moving toward more effective interaction, albeit slowly. The educational programs met with mixed reviews. Some administrators felt that they were not very successful and had mediocre attendance with more nurses participating than physicians. Moreover, meetings at a specific hospital were far better attended by the host hospital staff than by others, though one of the purposes was interhospital communication. The administrators felt that the committees were fairly successful, but there had been no attempt to develop aftercare. Cooperation among the urban four had probably improved, but little else had been achieved. However, the committee had facilitated planning and had created an atmosphere conducive to further planning. The administrators were concerned about the future of the CCA and felt that it might die after the end of the grant or become merely an educational cooperative program.

THE RURAL FIVE
HOSPITALS' VIEWS

It must be noted that some history of association and collaboration preceded the CCA, and there had been some shifts in the referral patterns predating the CCA as the needs for specialized care grew.

The primary reason for joining the CCA was in most cases a question of self-defense. Since no financial commitment was asked, it seemed logical to join rather than to possibly be at a disadvantage by not joining. A secondary reason was that of improving cancer care at the regional level or getting more care where it was needed.

The rural five had been members of the CCA for only a short time so it was difficult for them to evaluate its role since most of the time had been occupied with organizational issues. Some still felt that they should have been asked to join at the outset, but others felt that the elapsed time was necessary to begin the organizational process, and thus they experienced no sense of exclusion although they resented the lack of information about early activities. In fact, those who had feelings of exclusion were reinforced in their concerns when the initial recommendation for voting on the board was that they would have only one vote apiece while the four initial institutions would continue to have one for each representative, that is, three votes. The reasons for this recommendation seemed to have resulted from the original institutions' fear of an unwieldy decision process and of being outvoted. The result was that the rural hospitals felt excluded and alienated from the original institutions. While the voting situation was eventually corrected, the rural five also felt that the urban four, with little respect for the quality of care available at the rural hospitals, viewed them as simply sources of patients. Many people on the rural five staffs commented that their medical staffs certainly had little or no time to express their views. While they shared many views, those hospitals with more recently appointed administrators, those with tougher administrators, those farthest away from the town, and those with least to lose by any reallocation of resources were least concerned with the amount of participation they were allowed on the CCA. So while some members felt that their fears were justified, others felt that the voting issue was not divisive but rather intended to facilitate organizational development and that the others' paranoia was a function of personalities rather than of real events.

The central tumor registry was a positive factor, although it was not clear what benefits the institutions expected as a result of having a central registry. Since several institutions already had their own registries, it seemed clear that they could provide data to review physician performance should they choose to do so. It would appear that the potential benefit of the central tumor registry was less important than the fact that its establishment could not be argued about, was not likely to occur in the immediate future, would not affect the internal operations of member institutions, and would not at least for the time being require commitment in the form of funding. Some felt, however, that its development was proceeding too slowly.

Potential benefits might be derived from a consultation service, particularly if it took the form of education or sessions performed by circuit-riding specialists who would see patients in situ and thus reduce patient loss to other institutions.

All of the rural five agreed that education was a worthwhile goal. They felt that the major thrust should be in coordinating the individual hospital efforts and in facilitating the visits of consultants to the individual institutions to provide teaching sessions. Thus there was good reaction to the nursing programs so far developed. In addition, some hospital staff felt that the CCA should be a center for the development of new ideas and technology and their dissemination through the educational process. Others felt that they might be involved in research protocols that would provide them with the benefits of new technologies as well as educating them to new drugs.

All five hospitals seemed to agree that the CCA could well facilitate access to specialized high technology since the educational programs and organizational meetings would promote increased communications and therefore make it easier to know what was going on and to whom one might send patients.

The development of guidelines regarding screening or diagnostic or treatment standards were generally commended. The rural five would not necessarily have proposed these as high-priority goals, but they felt that the standards were worthwhile activities since somebody else was developing them. However, the hospital staffs were more enthusiastic about the diagnostic rather than the treatment standards since they felt that treatment varied widely. However, there was a clear consensus that while guidelines were good, they could not, in the interests of physician autonomy, be mandated and should be implemented only through an educational process in which they were made available to institutions and physicians. In any case, there was so much variation in treatments that the CCA could not really arrive at viable standards, and any standards they did set should simply be brought to the attention of physicians. Others felt that there was more available and needed in the way of sanctions than this rather passive approach, including the use of research protocols, as a distinct incentive for those who chose to adopt standards. A possible in-hospital procedure that some felt could be powerful and should be the means for sanction was the medical audit. Some of the hospitals' staff felt that bringing a doctor's behavior to public attention would in itself be a sufficient deterrent, and that eventually hospitals would have the options of either publishing survival figures or, in extreme cases, withholding hospital privileges. One doctor's suggestion was that it would be easy to make standards mandatory by simply requiring them to be part of the legal patient record. There was a general consensus against mandatory implementation of standards but a recognition that some mechanisms would be invoked.

The rural five were most concerned about the CCA's mandating standards such as saying who should specialize, that is, that *A* hospitals should do certain procedures, *B* hospitals less complex procedures, and *C* hospitals the most routine procedures. As far as the rural five were concerned, that was HSA business and should always be voluntary. It was acknowledged that in those hospitals that performed only oncology surgery, a patient was more likely to receive surgery than an alternative form of treatment through the existing referral process. Some staff felt that the addition of visiting medical oncologists would restore the balance somewhat, although it would not be as good as having the resources within the hospital. If administrators felt they were in conflict with the decisions of the CCA, they would inevitably take the hospitals' side. The existence of the CCA should not stop physicians from referring patients outside the CCA hospitals should they wish to do so. There was distinct hostility toward the notion that the CCA might decide on the basis of volume that, for example, surgical cases should be referred to oncology surgical specialists who saw such patients in sufficient numbers to guarantee high quality of care rather than to the general surgeon who seldom treated a cancer patient and who was thus not acquainted with the state-of-the-art surgical procedures.

It was clear that the rural five sincerely felt that they had distinct roles to play within the CCA and that they should not simply be regarded as consumers of the resources supplied by the urban four. While they acknowledged their primary-care role, they felt that they had some degree of specialized capability that should not be ignored. They also felt that standards were reasonable but should not be imposed. The CCA should not act as a policeforce but should add to the hospitals' capabilities. In addition, there was a clear feeling that while they joined to influence the CCA, they were to some degree at the mercy of the CCA also.

DEVELOPMENT OF THE CANCER COLLABORATION ASSOCIATION

Many CCA members felt that the CCA had to settle down to actually accomplishing something. If it continued to pursue those relatively trivial activities that were unthreatening but marginally useful, then at the critical point where the federal dollar ran out and the local dollar had to take over, most of the activities would not been seen to be worth funding either by the member institutions or by the community agencies. On the other hand, if more important activities were engaged in such as developing community programs or facing some of the dilemmas of reallocating resources and upgrading quality of care by more than exhortation, then the CCA ran a risk of losing some of its members who might be threatened by activities of this sort. Either way, there was a risk. It should be noted that there was a risk in being conservative as well as in moving toward confronting critical issues, but any risk involved leadership, and the CCA staff at the time of the study were not in this role, while the member institutions seemed unprepared to take on anything.

Another issue was the hospital-oriented focus of the CCA, which started with four major acute-care hospitals and extended to a further five. The CCA did not include any community-care institutions. It had focused exclusively on hospital-oriented care and, in particular, physician and professional care. Yet it could be argued that the major needs for the cancer patient were not in the area of technical care, for even the least sophisticated of the regional hospitals probably provided a reasonable quality of cancer care compared with some areas of the country. There might well be a much greater need for attention to the psychological and social aspects of patient and family functioning in cancer. Yet nothing was known about patient needs from the patient and community themselves, for no one had yet studied this, as though the medical system were perfectly satisfied that it knew what its patients needed.

In the same way that there had been little attention from the CCA to health care institutions outside acute care, there had been little attention to the range of community agencies with whom the CCA might work to augment its influence, perhaps again a reflection of the acute-care hospital orientation of all concerned. Possibly a more profound issue was that so far, little attention had been paid to the decision-making process other than a concern with proliferating bureaucracy. In fact, the size of the decision-making group, the board, at this time approached twenty-nine people. Was the board, and in particular voting as a method, an appropriate mechanism for reaching critical decisions? When decisions were made without all member institutions being present, nonparticipating institutions could effectively avoid commitment by avoiding decision making. Should there be an executive group with delegated power? Should there be decision only by consensus? Did, in fact, the committees make decisions (or should they have), and did the board, as the larger senate, simply ratify what had already been decided? What was the point of making decisions in the board arena when apparently the hospitals were disposed to ignore them when it came to implementing them? It seemed that many of the screening guidelines had been overwhelmed in a maze of bureaucracy, and there was very little evidence of implementation. It was difficult to assess whether the hospitals didn't follow through because of inertia or because the approach was somewhat unpopular.

Moreover, it was not clear whether the CCA was meant to be hierarchical—that is, a superior decision-making body that could impose its decisions upon its member institutions—or whether it was meant to be a loose conglomeration of members who might or might not choose to adhere to its decisions. It was certain that the CCA maintained and respected the sovereignties of the member institutions, but this did not mean that the CCA had to be without teeth.

In the realm of developing a sense of purpose, what about

commitment on the part of the member institutions of the CCA? There was a distinction between the reasons for joining and purpose. The fact that the original four hospitals had reasons for joining and developed a particular purpose did not mean that the rural five or even the urban four institutions were still committed to this original purpose. An important aspect of commitment is the development of a decision-making process that binds the actions of member institutions to whatever the CCA has determined. Evidence suggested that in fact this power had not yet been developed. What was clear was that the member hospitals, at least as far as the rural five were concerned, had not yet come to grips with what their existing roles were within the CCA, not had they come to grips with the CCA as a potential centralized source of decision making to which they might become subject. They essentially saw it more as a cow they could milk for certain purposes.

It was also not clear whether the CCA saw itself as a planning body, an organizational body, or an educational body. The member institutions, especially the rural five, highly valued the educational activities of the CCA because these were least threatening, and they also appeared to value the capability of the CCA for facilitating their planning, especially in conflict situations involving high technology. It was less clear whether the CCA had the organizational capacity to help in conflict resolution rather than simply to endorse certain activities as opposed to others. In other words, could the CCA not only plan programs but also encourage individual members to put them on either separately or in association? The future of the CCA would be in question at that point at which the member institutions had to participate financially and decide what they would choose to pay for. While all valued the centralized information capability of the tumor registry, it was not clear whether they would in fact be prepared to pay for it. They might, however, pay for some additional consultation visits. It was clear that the community would pay only for visible community programs that were non-hospital oriented, and it felt strongly that the hospitals should pay for their own internal activities such as professional education, which the CCA had focused heavily on.

The hospitals found it difficult to reconcile their interests with those of the CCA. One of the stated goals of the CCA was to improve the quality of care through the development of standards. Yet the CCA staff and the hospitals appeared to be adamant that these should be part of an educational process in which the hospitals would largely be left to, or encouraged to, implement whatever standards were developed. In reality, it was likely that good physicians would already be working to standards, and poor physicians would ignore any that were developed. Hospitals were extremely variable in the extent to which they possessed and implemented peer review. While some of the rural hospitals were quite aggressive in this respect and would use standards and implement them either through the peer-review mechanism or through making them part of the medical record, others were reluctant to do so. It was already clear that the hospitals were largely dragging their feet in circulating, let alone implementing, standards. Was this because they did not feel a part of their development, because they did not value them, or because they recognized the potential dangers should the CCA demand mandatory implementation? It was not at all clear that in this and other respects that there was any commitment on the part of the member institutions to the actions of the CCA or the CCA staff.

This situation was complicated because even if the CCA felt that it was important to mandate certain actions, what sanctions or incentives were available to it to ensure the adherence of member institutions? Certainly the CCA could require each member institution to use its internal mechanisms to implement commonly agreed-upon goals. But there were other incentives and sanctions that had not been used such as making available research protocols. The existing sanctions and incentives included peer review, legalizing the patient record, educational disapproval, and keeping or losing referrals. The Professional Standards Review Organization (PSRO) possessed the means, which it was not apparently prepared to use, to withhold payment if standards were not met, and, in fact, the CCA members seemed to feel that PSRO should be the policeman. While there apparently existed a mechanism for doing this, the PSRO representatives seemed to be very disinclined to invoke this except as a last resort. In other words, they were not willing to be policemen. Attention needed to be paid to how action could be implemented through sanctions and incentives.

Finally a caution: It is inappropriate and unfair to discuss significant program achievements given that only two years have passed since CCA began; the focus of this story is organizational process at the early stages of collaboration.

Chapter 7

The South Middlesex Hospital Association, Inc.

HISTORICAL PERSPECTIVES

The South Middlesex Hospital Association (SMHA) was developed in 1975 to "promote collaborative solutions to common problem areas." The association presently comprises five acute-care hospitals and two chronic/rehabilitation facilities. Six of these are located in two municipalities—Cambridge and Somerville, Massachusetts—which are immediately adjacent to the city of Boston. Included are a county hospital, two religious-affiliated hospitals, one small general hospital, and three larger community hospitals, two of which have teaching affiliations with Harvard Medical School.

When the association was originally formed, it was recognized that the diversity of the types of care the hospitals offered would bring advantages as well as disadvantages, so some of the hospitals are in chronic-care while others are acute-care facilities, and size, as indicated by variation in the net revenues of the various hospitals, ranges from small to large (Table 7.1). While the service area of the association's hospitals has definable geographic limits, its proximity to Boston leads to the association hospitals' competing with the Boston hospitals.

The data presented here were gathered in 1977 and hence do not reflect the present status of the South Middlesex Hospital Association.

Table 7-1. SMHA Hospital Characteristics (Fiscal Year 1978)

Year: 1977	Number of Beds	Number of Yearly Inpatient Admissions	Net Revenues[a]	Patient Services	Teaching
Mt. Auburn	300	9,534	$32,000,000	Full range of general and specialities	Yes: Harvard
Cambridge City	190	6,910	14,900,000	Full range of general	Yes: Harvard
Central	105	2,360	4,300,000	No pediatrics	No
Youville	305	559	13,000,000	Rehabilitation and chronic disease	No
Sancta Maria	150	4,243	8,500,000	Partial range of general	No
Somerville	140	4,752	9,900,000	Partial range of general	Yes: Tufts
Middlesex County	170	N.A.	5,000,000	Rehabilitation and chronic disease	No

[a]Net revenues equal gross patient revenues minus (1) contractual allowances, (2) free care, and (3) provision for uncollectable accounts.

The stated goals of the association are:

1. To improve regional health care and health-care delivery by means of collaborative planning.
2. To coordinate hospital planning and hospital activities.
3. To minimize health care costs.
4. To coordinate the efforts of its members to provide and arrange for the diagnosis and treatment of disease and for continuity of care.
5. To use the resources, equipment, and facilities of the member institutions efficiently.
6. To improve the quality of educational programs and of patient care.

The executive director of Mt. Auburn Hospital, one of the two largest hospitals in the association, is responsible for the development of the SMHA and was its first president. Before coming to Mt. Auburn Hospital, he had accumulated considerable experience in running a consortium in another city. He was recruited by the Mt. Auburn Hospital trustees because of this experience.

He was surprised at the lack of communication between the Cambridge area hospitals as compared with those in his previous experience. Soon after he arrived, he designed an organizational structure intended to improve relationships among the eventual member institutions. As a way of introducing himself to his colleagues in the community, he made a personal visit to each of the chief executive officers to determine the extent to which they were interested in his proposal. He did in fact receive an initial expression of interest from the community that contrasted with an unsuccessful earlier attempt to bring the hospitals together several years before.

Early on it was realized that the board of the association could not give policy direction to the organization or deal with substantive issues regarding clinical decision making unless hospital trustees and physicians were represented on the board. Administrators, trustees, and physicians all had to be involved from the outset if they were to take the association seriously. Consequently, the board of the association was, and still is, composed of three representatives (one of each category) from each of the seven hospitals, totaling twenty-one voting members. The physician representatives are usually the presidents of the medical staffs or the chairmen of the medical staff executive committees. The trustees tend to be the chairmen of the boards.

The first year was spent in getting acquainted and in defining the purposes of the consortium more clearly. While the administrators seemed to understand what the consortium was all about, the trustees and physicians apparently had little background and understanding of what "working together" meant. They had no personal knowledge about either clinical or functional joint planning, and they had nothing in their backgrounds to prepare them for this job.

Some physicians and others felt that the association developed because the hospitals involved thought they needed a common response to increasing governmental regulations, especially the HSA. However, at the same time there was also a great deal of fear on the part of the institutions toward one another.

During the second year of the association's development, an executive director, Alan Nichols, was selected, and the board meetings were more formally organized. Alan Nichols had been doing research for the Health Planning Council (HPC) for Greater Boston and had written a study of maternity care in greater Boston, which recommended that Mt. Auburn and Cambridge Hospitals explore the feasibility of either closing one of their units or merging them. His planning knowledge and contacts tended to confirm the association's rationale of counterplanning. The difficulty of reconciling the association's diversity led Nichols to visit each hospital at some length to get acquainted with it and its representatives. He made many contacts and tried to elicit views as to the purpose of the association, current problem areas, and personal priorities:

> What I was looking for, at least initially, was to find out who the leaders were on my board because it would be through these people that I would make recommendations and have them present my ideas at the board meetings, rather than make them directly. My experience before I got involved with this multi-organizational system was pretty much research and a little administration, but mostly research; so I really was not aware of the nuances of how you play the ego or power game, whom you talk to and whose toes you step and don't step on, and whom you avoid. It really took me about five months of talking to people to learn who the significant actors were and which individuals really had respect from the entire board.

Alan Nichols believes that the Mt. Auburn director is still the major conceptualizer and systems thinker in the association. Most of the others are more interested in the plans of neighboring institutions rather than regional health care. Both Nichols and he agree that even a hospital consortium is too narrow. Nichols says:

> We have a nursing home representative who is also a vice president of the board of directors of the Health Planning Council on one of our subcommittees, our policy trustees committee, and essentially that is because of my emphasis too that multi-institutional arrangements can't involve just hospitals. You're going to be using nursing homes as major referral areas. If you're using Harvard Community Health Plan that sends it patients all over the place, you've got to involve them in the system! It's just a question of process. The ultimate goal is to have many units tied into a multi-institutional network. But my hospitals even now don't have their act together and there is no way I want to upset the applecart by trying to put nursing home or HMO representatives into major roles in my board meeting. That is why I will ease the Harvard Community Health Plan into our medical committee. It will be brought up at a board meeting and then it will be discussed at a future medical committee meeting. It is

just a question of time. In the entire Association, the physicians are the most conservative, the most resistant to any type of real variation and change. But without physicians, the Association is going to fall apart. They are the key to the whole thing and the group that has been least involved in the Association in the past year and a half.

STRUCTURE

Each hospital was asked to send the president of its board of trustees, the president of the medical staff, and the director to participate in the monthly executive board meetings of the association. Attendance was variable, although at least one representative from each hospital usually attended the meetings on a fairly regular basis. Most consistent were the hospital administrators. Alan Nichols made up the agendas for the meetings and tried also to meet with each hospital member individually on a monthly basis.

During the first year the members took turns making presentations to the board on the current and future status of their institutions and reported on the progress being made by the different committees and subcommittees. In addition, guest speakers were invited occasionally to address the board on various issues, e.g., federal, state, and local aspects of the new health-planning legislation.

About a year after the board meetings were first established, the group met to discuss the current and future status of the association. Questions were raised as to the need for the association and whether it represented a good investment of time. The members agreed that given Public Law 93-641, the association enabled them to influence the system rather than simply being dictated to by the newly developed Health Systems Agency. The members agreed that a primary goal of the SMHA was to improve the regional health care delivery system in a collaborative fashion, and the secondary goal was to increase the operational efficiency of the member hospitals via shared services.

Many association members expressed concern over the fact that physicians had not been actively involved in the association during its first year, fearing that their distance could easily become criticism or even hostility. It was suggested that the physician representatives be elected by the president of the medical staff or by the medical staff executive committee of each of the member hospitals.

In addition, it was noted that in order to improve health care delivery in the region, it would be necessary to compare three- and five-year plans as stated in the new health-planning legislation. It was decided that the association would develop a common format for presenting such plans. Given the new federal and state legislation regarding Certificate of Need regulations and criteria, the board members agreed that it was absolutely essential for the participating hospitals to share in their short- and long-range plans with each other, and that the physicians should be the group most involved with this endeavor.

This was a time when the future of the association seemed to be at stake. Finally, three committees—policy, medical, and management—were set up, and the board delegated major responsibilities to them. The medical committee members drew up a list of key issues, decided priorities, and set up a series of task forces, one for each topic, in part as a way of involving more doctors. Theoretically, membership in any committee could consist of any board member—trustee, physician, or administrator—but as it turned out, habit won, and trustees went to the policy committee, physicians to the medical committee, and administrators to the management committee.

The medical committee did have for a short time one non-physician from Somerville Hospital. Although an administrator, he was very interested in and knowledgeable about medical matters, but the physicians asked him to leave the committee, and Somerville replaced him with a physician. Obviously the medical committee lost his administrative expertise.

Alan Nichols submitted a proposal outlining the activities that each of the three committees would handle. The committees accepted his proposal. He described the three committees as follows:

> The policy committee consists of trustees and deals with broad issues. It is this committee which works on the review and amendment of the bylaws and monitors the overall mission and progress of the Association. The medical committee deals with clinical and medical issues which have effects over a much longer span of time; the management committee is concerned with short-term administrative cost-savings ventures for the Association.

Policy Committee

Once an issue is discussed and a bylaw has been cleared by the policy committee, the entire SMHA board has to clear it; then it has to be approved by the board of each member hospital. Policy statements are voted on in the policy committee but do not necessarily have an effect because the boards of the individual hospitals retain their institutional autonomy. Its objective is to work on the bylaws and to make general policy statements. One of its jobs is to make the boards of the various member hospitals aware that the consortium exists. Many of the boards are not aware of the SMHA, and the policy committee according to some members has not done very much about it. The policy committee, according to one member, does not really have the brain power to decide on issues like "who should have this or that service."

Medical Committee

The medical committee is chaired by a radiologist from Mt. Auburn Hospital, who is one of the leaders of the SMHA.

The key issues on the medical committee agenda have included: chronic disease and cancer care; medical education; delineation of staff privileges; combining Ob/Gyn and pediatric resources; relationships with the medical schools; CAT scanner acquisition; the role of the hospitals in the community-based primary-care satellite clinics and emergency medical care.

The physicians have generally been involved only in those areas that directly concern their hospitals, e.g., Middlesex County's physician representative having been involved only with the chronic-disease and cancer-care task forces. The medical education task force involves only the three teaching hospitals.

An administrator commented on his expulsion:

The basic reason was that doctors were unwilling to talk frankly about the business of medicine in the presence of a layman. I could have made useful contributions on issues of medical care. But lots of issues that they wanted to discuss had to do with the business of medicine in Cambridge, and there is some friction between physicians in Cambridge over staff privileges.

A physician member on the medical committee justified the committee's actions:

To the physicians, including a non-physician seemed to be dysfunctional, and the physicians voted to exclude the non-physician from the medical committee. This was done more from an organizational rather than a personal point of view, but it is interpreted the other way around. A group of just physicians can bring more skills to look at medical issues. The whole problem was that the board was too unspecific in charging the various committees with particular responsibilities; also, it did not specify the manner in which these committees would be constructed. The board could have said that the medical committee membership would be

2 + 2 + 2, or that all six would be physicians; in either case, no bad feelings would have been formed because of an administrator being asked to leave the medical committee.

If the medical committee consisted of 2 + 2 + 2 members, we would be doing nothing different from what goes on at board meetings. There would thus be duplication of time and effort. Further, it is not that I, as a physician, am not interested in working with administrators. If that were so, I would not be attending the board meetings at all. It is just that the medical committee with its physician membership is a more appropriate setting to discuss specific medical issues.

Management Committee

The management committee has seven administrators on it. They are all overly committed, so Alan Nichols until recently did the majority of the background work and then left it to them to say yes or no. His first priority is his work with the management committee.

In addition to the committees, Nichols developed several allied organizations consisting of members of each hospital in the areas of medical records, administration, nursing directors, pharmacy directors, personnel, education directors, emergency medical service, purchasing and material management, and social service directors. Members of these organizations get together periodically to get to know one another and discuss mutual problems and concerns and to try to work together on various projects.

INSTITUTIONS: ROLES AND VIEWS

Mt. Auburn Hospital

Mt. Auburn Hospital is a 300-bed, voluntary, nonprofit teaching hospital, which provides general medical, surgical, obstetrics and gynecology, pediatrics, and psychiatric care to the surrounding communities. The hospital was set up in 1870 by a special act of the state legislature. Most chiefs of service are located in the geographic vicinity on a full-time basis. Many subspecialty chiefs are also similarly geographically located on a full-time basis. There are fifty-two house physicians.

The hospital provides postgraduate training to Harvard Medical School students, particularly through a surgical residency. Many undergraduates from Harvard, Tufts, and Boston University obtain some of their clinical experience at Mt. Auburn. If the association institutions were to be ranked in terms of power, Mt. Auburn would unquestionably top the list as it is the wealthiest, the most aggressive, the most powerful, and according to many, the best hospital in terms of general medical care.

A radiologist at Mt. Auburn, considered to be one of the more influential physicians in the area and a board member of the association, noted that many of the physicians in the area feared the association and that in general, physicians do not get involved in the management of their own hospitals because they are busy with their medical work and own medical organizations. His view is that the association has dealt with easy, nonthreatening issues only, e.g., the standardization of record keeping, coordination of equipment and emergency care, and joint purchases. The members have not been willing to bring up substantive issues. He suggests that a consortium tends to develop very slowly and goes through a succession of stages: At the first stage, the formal association is set up; at the second stage, the member institutions start making tangible monetary contributions to the association; and at the third stage, the members agree to meet and talk over problems that are least threatening to the autonomy of each member institution. The third stage is where he believes the SMHA is presently.

A senior administrator at Mt. Auburn Hospital recognizes that this larger and more sophisticated hospital is constantly being accused of trying to co-opt the association and that there has not been complete success in reducing that fear. In some respects, in fact, Mt. Auburn has less to gain from the association than the other hospitals, but it would be willing to support joint ventures over solo efforts even if they cost more because it was prepared to subordinate its interests for the good of the association. There was, for example, one instance when the board of trustees of Mt. Auburn extended hospital privileges to outside MDs to admit their patients for radiation therapy when it was mutually decided between the radiation therapist and the outside MD that such treatment was necessary. The physician was allowed to admit and follow the patient during the entire course of radiation therapy and therefore did not worry about losing his patient. On another occasion, Mt. Auburn submitted a Certificate of Need application for a CAT scanner to serve all the association hospitals, offering assurances that each hospital would have guaranteed time on the machine, emergency cases would be covered within two hours, and Mt. Auburn would provide coverage on a twenty-four-hour, seven-day-per-week basis.

This administrator agrees that the association is in a transitional phase and is slowly moving from insignificant to significant issues.

This process has taken longer than he had anticipated, as some of the hospitals are still pretty much at the point where they were when they originally joined the association. This lack of progress is not perhaps surprising since the major reason for their membership in the SMHA was the fear that they would be sabotaged by the other hospitals if they were not involved and were not kept informed of what their counterparts were doing. Paranoia often motivates membership in a consortium. The association is now at the point where its members are beginning to coordinate their efforts on less important issues, such as collection of bad debts and repair services for biomedical equipment. Major issues such as allocation and regionalization of services are not yet being addressed seriously. Potential cost savings is not a powerful reason for the hospitals to collaborate because current federal legislation does not provide any positive or negative financial incentives to collaborating institutions. Even if the seven hospitals could accomplish area-wide planning and were able to save a substantial amount of money, it would not be returned to them.

Cambridge City Hospital

Cambridge City Hospital is a 210-bed acute-care municipal and Harvard teaching facility. A senior administrator there believes that services such as obstetrics, pediatrics, psychiatry, emergency room, and neighborhood health centers are a major concern among the member hospitals because any imposed redistribution of services can lead to the "domino effect" in which closing an obstetrical service, for example, can in turn cut off the flow of other types of patients, such as pediatrics.

One of the major problems facing Cambridge City Hospital is that it has never really had a good strong board. It does not have any planning staff. There are political problems and problems with the public image of the hospital. The hospital does not spend any money on public relations, although a senior administrator there feels it should. Thus the clientele consists of poor patients, alcoholics, drug addicts, and the neurotic illnesses of the poor; middle-class citizens do not think it is a good hospital in spite of its excellent staff.

The relationship between Cambridge City Hospital and Mt. Auburn Hospital is not good. Mt. Auburn serves the middle class, spends an enormous amount of money on public relations, and has an excellent board. Both Mt. Auburn and Cambridge City are Harvard teaching hospitals, and they compete for the same money—much of which comes from the medical school budget—and for teaching programs, especially with regard to primary-care and family-practice programs. Mt. Auburn Hospital has the resources, and Cambridge City has the patient population. The Harvard Community Health Plan (Cambridge Center) is another and new competitor since it does not have its own hospital and must use the other hospitals in the area when patient hospitalization is required.

The administrator would like to see a master plan developed that would determine what services were needed and what the optimal resource configuration would be. He sees accessibility, acceptability, cost effectiveness, and teaching as key issues. Since the Cambridge area is very overbedded, he would like to see the city-run neighborhood health centers be responsible for the primary care delivered in the area. Mt. Auburn should concentrate on secondary-care delivery, and the Massachusetts General Hospital should be responsible for all the tertiary care delivered to the patients in the area. Extended care should be delivered by nursing homes, and mental health care should be delivered by neighborhood health centers and the Sancta Maria Hospital. The other institutions should be closed or converted to other uses. Cambridge City Hospital could then become the psychiatric, drug addiction, and alcoholic facility for the Cambridge and Somerville areas and could then attract specialized research oriented staff people.

He sees little financial incentive to the city from the cost savings of rationalizing health services. The city of Cambridge is going to have to make a decision as to how much of a financial load it wants to carry because it is a myth that the City Hospital can be run at breakeven since nearly half the patients have no insurance coverage.

Central Hospital

Central Hospital is a 127-bed, for-profit hospital owned by one man. Of the 127 beds, 20 are for psychiatric care, 16 are for alcohol and drug detoxification, and the remainder are for medical and surgical care. The hospital has an emergency room and an outpatient department with a number of clinics, for example, geriatric, pediatric, well-baby, and ophthalmology.

A senior physician at Central believes that the SMHA is a good concept, although he has not been personally involved in it since he is not seeking anything from the association, nor is he being paid to attend the medical committees. He believes that the only physicians who attend the meetings are the ones being paid to attend them or the ones having some interests to protect. In another instance, a hospital's service is in danger of being closed down, so its physicians attend the meetings on their own time to protect their personal interests.

An administrator thought that Central Hospital joined the association with the understanding that member institutions would help each other in such areas as joint purchasing, which would provide access to resources that single hospitals could not afford. He considers it an interesting phenomenon that within the association there is not one institution or one individual who thinks about what is best for the community before considering what is best for himself or his institution. The major problem currently facing Central Hospital is its uncertainty about its future survival. Somerville Hospital wants to see Central Hospital closed down so that it can get extra beds, but Sancta Maria Hospital, in turn, is determined to make sure that Somerville Hospital does not get a Certificate of Need if Somerville should make application for such additional beds. The administrator sees Cambridge City and Mt. Auburn Hospitals fighting over a CAT scanner, which neither of them, in his opinion, needs.

Youville Hospital

Youville Hospital is a 305-bed chronic-disease rehabilitation facility. It was founded by the Grey Nuns in 1890 and for a long time was a long-stay chronic-disease hospital, essentially for the terminally ill. The rehabilitation center was built in the 1950s. Youville Hospital is currently in the process of replacing their fifty-year-old building with a new one because of safety standards. They plan to maintain the current staff and ancillary services. The president of the Youville board of directors is vice-president of SMHA.

One of the administrators believes that there are no real alternatives to the kind of care that Youville supplies.

He believes that the association is concerned with the total delivery of health care and that Youville has a clear role to play. Normally hospitals have a tendency to become self-absorbed in their own area of expertise, and the association has given him the opportunity to understand better the problems of acute-care institutions, although he also feels that they should involve nursing homes. He echoes other's sentiments about physicians who seem to want to protect their interests as much as possible, pay only lip service to costs, and expect everyone except themselves to avoid duplication of services.

Middlesex County Hospital

Middlesex County Hospital is a 170-bed county hospital licensed for chronic-disease and tuberculosis care. Over 100 of the beds are allocated for chronic disease, 22 for tuberculosis, 9 for spinal cord injury, and 35 for alcohol detoxification. The philosophy of the hospital is to respond to the county's needs for health services for severely disabled people. It concentrates on rehabilitation as well as the medical care needs of the patient population. It is a public hospital, cares for patients in primarily the older age groups, and is funded largely by third-party reimbursement—e.g., Medicaid and Medicare—with but little private insurance.

Middlesex County was a tuberculosis hospital at the time the association was being formed, and it was losing clientele quite rapidly. When the present incumbent became administrator, the hospital was beginning to diversify into chronic care and had been running a deficit for seven years. The year he joined, there was a deficit of $3.5 million. It was not clear either to Middlesex County staff or to outsiders as to whether there was a viable role for such a facility in the South Middlesex area. Middlesex County Hospital is actually closer to another consortium with which, however, it has nothing in common.

A Middlesex County Hospital administrator feels that Youville may have a large percentage of nursing home patients and that the area may not need it as a hospital. They have currently applied for a CON to renovate their beds, and sooner or later, he will be asked to endorse this application. When this happens, it will pose a problem for him.

The Middlesex County Hospital has two Certificate of Need applications pending. One is for an alcoholic residency program, and the other is for $500,000 worth of capital improvements. The administrator maintains that the fate of these applications is affected by the Department of Health's image of chronic-care hospitals. The cost per day per bed in a chronic-disease hospital is about twice that of a nursing home. The Department of Public Health is in a dilemma over how to deal with this situation. The administrator suggested to the department that they periodically review all chronic-disease hospitals for appropriateness of patient care. This type of review was completed at Middlesex. According to the administrator, the department concluded that 81 percent of the patients at Middlesex were placed there appropriately. The hospital had attempted to place the remaining 19 percent in level II nursing homes but had been unsuccessful.

On the other hand, the administrator believes that less than a quarter of Youville Hospital's patients may be appropriately placed there, and so all the Youville patients could be accommodated at the Middlesex County Hospital.

Another problem facing the hospital is the issue of Medicare reimbursement. Under current regulations, Medicare reimbursement is generally made only to acute-care hospitals or to nursing homes. Reimbursement to chronic-disease hospitals is made on a case-by-case basis only. According to the proposed regulations, Medicare reimbursement would be denied to any hospital with more than 10 percent inappropriately placed patients. Some hospital representatives have found their experience in the association not unmixed, and they share others' concerns with the rampant parochialism.

One physician was asked to attend the association meetings as one of the hospital's representatives. Initially, he attended very regularly, but as he found other MDs absenting themselves and the meetings to be frustrating and largely administrative in nature, his attendance dropped off. He still feels it is very important for the association to succeed and that other physicians think the association has offered them an opportunity to share experiences with each other.

This physician's view of the goals of the association are:

1. To improve communication between the member institutions.
2. To get the member institutions to share services.
3. To get the member institutions to educate each other.
4. To find gaps in the existing health care delivery system.
5. Overall, to provide better health care delivery to the community.

Sancta Maria Hospital

Sancta Maria Hospital is a 150-bed acute medical and surgical care hospital with a 5-bed intensive and coronary care unit. It is a private nonprofit Catholic hospital.

An executive of Sancta Maria believes that the central purpose of the association is to be able to deal effectively with state and local agencies such as the HSA. He admits that the association is still suffering "growing pains" because of the continuing strife and predicts that it will take about five years or more to achieve the kind of power that other consortia, such as the Capital Area Health Consortium, have achieved. Because the association's first president was from Mt. Auburn Hospital, other board members were suspicious. He describes the role of executive director as being the person who keeps on top of everything that goes on within the association and the HSA and, in addition, does a lot of regional planning.

Somerville Hospital

Somerville Hospital is a 140-bed acute-care facility. It is really on the periphery of the association in all respects, including geographically. Somerville has little to give to the other hospitals, and little to gain from them. One hospital executive would have preferred an alternative grouping of hospitals in which it would have been the center rather than on the periphery. Because of its relationship to the other hospitals, Somerville tends to act as the referee. Many of the issues facing the association are irrelevant to Somerville. For example, the resolution of the issue regarding Ob/Gyn and pediatrics services will have no bearing on Somerville, as it has neither of those two types of facilities. The major advantage to Somerville and to the other hospitals, in his opinion, of belonging to the association is that the state health agencies perceive them as being a strong unified force.

VIEWS OF ADMINISTRATION
AND PHYSICIANS

Administrators and physicians were frank in assessing themselves and each other's roles and performance.

Administrators:

Administrators are concerned with their entire hospital, and do have a prejudiced view about how they want to come out in the end. But this prejudice is normal and understandable. The medical profession has its prejudices too, particularly in regard to specific services. Even this is understandable and acceptable. However, many trustees are biased too, and that clearly should not be so. I am impressed by the quality of the administrators in this area.

I think the administrators know the value of giving the Association a chance. But the physicians are very resistant to change because this kind of coordination is a new idea.

With doctors, the basic problem is one of interest and awareness. They are not properly advised about the medical system itself, not to speak of the problems of administering a hospital.

Physicians by and large are fairly uniform in their objections and resistance to the idea of a consortium. The administrators are generally well informed about the field of health care, but I do not like their code of ethics. The board of trustees, on the other hand, display an awesome ignorance of the health care field and tend to be the most protective about institutional prerogatives.

A lot depends upon the abilities of the physician representatives to take the agreements made in the consortium setting and sell them back to their own people. You have to be in two roles at the same time. If you become too much of an outsider, then nothing may happen. Thus, you have to remain a respected insider, while differing from the rest of your colleagues. Physicians have tremendous peer ties and a strong peer culture. This must always be taken into account. All that they are concerned about is teaching and patient exposure.

Physicians are by and large disorganized.

I'm sure that the administrators can change relatively easily, meaning that they can start thinking of regional rather than institutional interests without much trouble. The key bottleneck are physicians. They are the most lousy investors, and the most lousy managers of their own affairs. They live in a very narrow world where they do not have to establish priorities between program A and program B. At the same time, from my personal contact with some physicians whom I know very well, I know that many of them are usually so busy with their medical work that they don't have time to get involved either in the administration of their own hospitals or the SMHA. Of course there are some exceptions and here and there you do find some doctors who are very progressive.

Doctors are different. They are at least not shallow, and they have a much stronger ability to understand things conceptually and abstractly. I thus find that it is easier to deal with doctors and convert them than to do the same with administrators. I dread meeting the latter. If I were looking for a hospital administrator, I know who I would not hire—somebody who is a member of SMHA and/or somebody with a degree in hospital administration.

Agreement from medical men and administrators is needed before implementation can take place. If physicians are not involved in the study process, they will always say that they were not involved and will thus not take any responsibility for the results. If physicians are going to accept a decision as their own, they have got to participate in the decision making process from the beginning. They have to be a party to it. It is the same thing with the board of trustees of the member institutions. They make policy decisions for the individual hospitals and thus have to be there from the very outset. Managers cannot do it by themselves.

Physicians:

The executive director should be known and respected. He should be reliable and trustworthy. He should be somebody who can be a leading figure in suggesting and responding to each hospital's needs and suggestions. The performance of the current executive director is not optimal.

Trustees have a very low level of involvement. The administrators are the most involved, but their involvement is not as significant or important as the involvement of physicians.

There need to be more opportunities for the physicians to understand each other. It would help if there was a better data base on who each physician is, what his role at each hospital is, and the kind of services that each hospital provides. I remember that during the early days of the consortium some data on each hospital had been distributed to the other hospitals. However, since the administrators had initiated that idea, the data was primarily administrative and fiscal, and therefore was not of interest to us. Ideally, if data regarding medical services were available properly, the consortium setup would encourage a matching of strengths and weaknesses.

The effectiveness of the role of executive director depends very much on the person and the role that the top people in the member institutions want to give him. For instance, within a hospital an administrator can be very easily over-run by a strong medical chief. The same kind of situation is reflected in the case of the executive director of a consortium.

Some of the physicians have been quite active in the consortium because of their long association with it and the region. By and large, they all feel that the consortium has offered them an opportunity to communicate with each other and has provided a good learning experience for them.

The loyalty and commitment of a physician is simultaneously to a number of bodies: to himself, to his profession, to his hospital, to his consortium, and so on. Consequently, he is a very busy individual. He therefore needs a strong reason to pick up an activity such as working on SMHA committees or task forces. The medical committee was set up in fall 1976 with just this purpose in mind, in order to help institutionalize the involvement of physicians in the Association. Prior to that, we had some ad-hoc task forces consisting of physicians—such as those on cancer, management, CAT scanning—and task forces consisting of some trustees and some physicians which just spun apart.

SOME MAJOR PROBLEMS

Competition is historically the American way of life. In addition to the minor feuds alluded to earlier, Cambridge Hospital and Mt. Auburn Hospital have differences over a number of other issues.

One contentious issue is the competition between the Ob/Gyn services at Cambridge City (which is Catholic in orientation) and Mt.

Auburn, which are of a very similar size. There is a third and somewhat larger service in Cambridge, the Harvard Community Health Plan-Harvard Health Service-M.I.T. Health Service, which currently uses Mt. Auburn's beds. With the exception of one doctor who is on the faculty at Tufts, all the other Cambridge services are affiliated with Harvard Medical School. Harvard does not initiate the appointment of chiefs but does have influence and may suggest candidates. Appointments are ratified by Cambridge's executive committee, city manager, and board of governors, who do not necessarily just go along with suggestions.

The main problem at Cambridge is a lack of research orientation among its service chiefs. While these service chiefs are involved in some teaching, many of them are not tenured professors at Harvard Medical School. Thus in spite of their long years of dedicated service, they have less prestige and less clout with the medical school. This fact creates many rifts between Cambridge City and Mt. Auburn. Also, the latter has expressed unwillingness to accord staff privileges to some of Cambridge City's doctors, particularly surgeons.

Because of the past close association of Mt. Auburn with Boston City, the Greene professorship of obstetrics initially was supposed to be placed at Mt. Auburn, as the money was raised and originally intended for Boston City. The goal was to develop a big service because both Mt. Auburn and Cambridge were too small to meet HSA standards for viability. But Harvard Medical School informed Mt. Auburn that the issue of the Greene professorship would be dropped until the matter of obstetrics in the city of Cambridge was more settled since it did not wish to side with one hospital over another. Harvard Medical School urged Mt. Auburn and Cambridge to get together with the help of outside experts.

One pediatrician at Cambridge believes obstetrics should be at Cambridge because it is the city hospital and it also cares for Somerville residents. He is obviously aware of the relationship of pediatrics to obstetrics.

Alan Nichols, responding to this connection also, commented:

> Mt. Auburn was considering closing its pediatric unit because it is less than half utilized but obviously the hospital does not want to do that unless there is some trade-off. I think that Mt. Auburn may eventually close its pediatric unit. Now I do not know what the trade-off will be. They are not going to close it and just give it away. They are looking for something. What I am trying to see is whether closure will be taken by Cambridge as an indication that they are going to get all of the pediatric load because their utilization is about 75%. Mt. Auburn's is 45%. Although I have good information on maternity and I am working with both hospitals on this

issue, I did not realize how ingrained the political structure was in Cambridge in terms of all the deals and in-fighting and everything that has to go on to get this done. I think that eventually you are going to have to have either a single unit or some type of combination. I really do not see both units surviving in the long run.

I believe that both hospitals are seeing whether they can get affiliations with the Harvard Community Health Plan so that the number of deliveries can be enhanced at one of the units. The Plan can essentially sit back and wait until the units of the hospitals come in and bargain, and it is an unfortunate situation. I have heard rumors that the Plan is thinking of setting up its own hospital.

Another dividing issue was which of the two hospitals should receive the CAT scanner that they both wanted. To some extent the decision of the consortium as to whose application to endorse seemed a foregone conclusion. Mt. Auburn had submitted its Certificate of Need application more than a year previously, while Cambridge had never submitted one. However, at the time a decision was to be made, Cambridge claimed that it was ready with a Certificate of Need application. To many it seemed more likely that Cambridge was showing interest in the CAT scanner issue primarily to improve its bargaining strength in the obstetrics unit case. At the board of directors meeting, a two-thirds majority was necessary for consortium support of Mt. Auburn's application. This was achieved. Cambridge City Hospital did not like the decision and so abstained from voting when the issue was put before the entire board. Although this increased animosity between Mt. Auburn and Cambridge City, some of the representatives felt that at least the association had reached the stage where the member hospitals could disagree with one another face to face.

The intense rivalry between Cambridge Hospital and Mt. Auburn has also extended to the development of surgical services at the respective hospitals. As increasing scarcity of resources becomes evident over time, development will become increasingly difficult, and so consequently both of them want to build up as many services as possible in the short run at their own institutions.

Of a more general nature is the problem of decision making. The representatives on the board seem to find it a difficult task to represent their institution and at the same time be a part of a team that is moving toward trying to manage the association. What seems to have evolved is a political forum that tends to distort the real issues in terms of any real objectivity. It has been suggested that noninstitutional representatives—for example, a health representative from the city of Cambridge or somebody from the local HSA—could participate and perhaps rise above the institutional parochialism. According to many members, if the association is to succeed, the members must start to put community objectives before institutional objectives and be responsive to the community's total needs and their institution's role within that framework. An example of neglecting this occurred when Mt. Auburn filed a grant application with the Robert Wood Johnson Foundation to obtain funding in order to establish primary-care units but failed to inform the other hospitals that it was doing so.

Another problem is related to the role of the executive director. Many seem to believe that an executive director of a multi-institutional system must know "when to put a stop to planning and when to tell people to start marching." He should be able to persuade, organize, facilitate, and brainstorm and help bring about consensus on important issues. Ideally, he should have had some hospital management experience and be a good organizational planner. Alan Nichols recognizes that one of the initial problems facing the association and for which he takes responsibility is that there was no effective organizational structure in the first year, and that in part this was due to his managerial inexperience, which he has now remedied.

The association has still to face the problem of credentials. As it stands now, a physician from one hospital cannot follow patients referred to another hospital. Neither the doctor nor the patient likes this kind of a situation. The major obstacle to that is that the hospitals do not all have the same standards and do not consider themselves equal.

Overall, a critical problem facing the association is the lack of trust on the part of the member hospitals toward one another. The hospitals formed the group for their protection rather than for regional planning. Many of the board members and staff of the various hospitals seem reluctant to share information with each other. Consequently, the association has to develop an agenda for purely organizational activities in the hope that coordination on the administrative issues will eventually lead to coordination on the more important ones. Many institutions are very concerned that Mt. Auburn, being large and strong, will get the jump with innovations over them. They see it as a threat. However, they feel that through the association, they can at least monitor, if not influence or control, its activities to some degree.

Perhaps it is this ambivalence that has led to the poor or erratic attendance at board meetings. Many believe that the association can work only if the members get to know and understand one another. This is difficult to achieve if the members do not attend the meetings on a regular basis.

> There is basically a lack of involvement. I myself stopped attending all their meetings several months ago. Before that, I remember that I would come all the way from Cape Cod on Friday morning at 8 a.m. to attend meetings at some hospital only to discover that only two other people were present. I got very frustrated and gave up.

For each of the hospitals except Mt. Auburn, attendance by administrators was better than by physicians or by trustees. Trustees averaged a 40-percent attendance rate, physicians averaged a 47-percent attendance rate, and administrators averaged a 70-percent attendance rate. Hospitals varied in attendance also. Trustee attendance at Cambridge Hospital was low, and administrator attendance high. Physician attendance at Mt. Auburn Hospital was very high, while administrators at Somerville and Sancta Maria attended very frequently. Youville Hospital representatives attended the least frequently across the board.

Committee attendance was quite varied. Only three hospitals, Cambridge, Mt. Auburn, and Sancta Maria, had representatives attend the management committee on a regular basis. The medical committee, however, had a high and consistent attendance rate.

Perhaps behind this poor attendance is the lack of incentives for collaboration apart from fear of the future. An administrator from Cambridge Hospital summed it up:

> To me it is crystal clear that institutions are not going to plan for themselves. They are self-serving; it is in the nature of the beast and it has got to be imposed. I think to regulate the imposition is just teasing the system; it has got to be like a guillotine; it has got to be sharp and swift.
>
> If you are not going to have external regulation, you have to have some incentives in the system for people to do something which is not immediately obviously in their own interest. The incentives at the moment seem to encourage hospitals to be as separate as possible because every hospital is trying to build up its own interest against the day that it may be forced to do something with other institutions. But it would be difficult to design a system that contains the incentives for people to do something different from what they are doing now. In the Cambridge situation, for example, if one wanted the key hospitals to get together and provide more efficient and cost-effective services, that might mean closing down some beds, losing some jobs, and the fact is that you may have an imposition

outside of regional planning areas. These do not correspond to political realities. The political realities are the cities, if one did in Cambridge what might be rational and ideal, i.e., cut some beds, improve services by reallocating, etc., there would be a loss of jobs and the Cambridge City would not tolerate this. There is no incentive except that of ideals for anybody to do anything about the Cambridge situation. It would mean losing jobs, losing patronage, losing power; sometimes at the expense of someone else, sometimes overall. The fact is that at the moment the only incentive to collaborate is when you get something else on top of what you have got. If that is the situation then people may collaborate a bit. They are not going to if they think that it involves losing something unless they get something else back which they value more.

PROGRESS AND PROSPECTS

In January 1977 a document entitled "Criteria for Information Sharing" was approved by the board. Its purpose was to provide policy and procedural guidelines for the exchange of information between the member hospitals. The criteria encouraged disclosure of planning activities and established some general boundaries within which such disclosure should occur to avoid repetition of some unpleasant surprises. The document specifically included definitions and policies and procedures regarding requests for data, grant applications, Certificate of Need applications, one- and five-year plans, and cooperative multi-institutional projects.

According to the executive director, the biggest accomplishment of the SMHA to date has been the release of each hospital's one-year plan.

In addition, the association has been successful in carrying out a number of low-key activities. For National Hospital Week, the association coordinated a week-long free clinic activity for area residents. Hospital disaster drills were carried out on a community-wide basis instead of on an individual hospital basis. The association has developed an in-service education program, a swine flu vaccination program, a credit collection, a data base, and a cancer management program. Additional activities include: more advice and sharing among the Cambridge Hospital and Central Hospital interns in psychiatry; patient transfer from one hospital to another; master list of work-study programs for each hospital; master list of emergency room equipment and cardiac monitors for sharing; biomedical engineering (advice on equipment by one firm for all the hospitals); three hospitals are considering using one security firm; sharing of an anesthesiologist between Cambridge and Central; shared emergency-room staffing between Mt. Auburn and Cambridge Hospitals (for one year only); presently working on restorative care, PT, OT, audiology (broker role for community); shared physician speakers bureau for medical education; smokers anonymous program; and EMS programs.

Other activities that Alan Nichols would like to see the association accomplish include: cardiopulmonary resuscitation training, the transfer of patients from one hospital to another, and the buying or leasing of vehicles for material and staff transfer between hospitals.

Many association members are not pleased with or optimistic about the achievements of the association. Some suggest that the association should start taking some concrete action to save money instead of being preoccupied with manuals, bylaws, committees, subcommittees, and surveys. They believe that they are just playing games and pursuing their own interests rather than those of the association. They feel the meetings are boring and repetitious and that nothing substantial has been accomplished. Many have predicted that the future success of the association will come about only through moral persuasion or if the inability to resolve disputes starts to hurt the individual members.

One physician suggests:

> These are tough issues. If we don't get our act together within a reasonable period of time, then a lot of our actions will be regulated by the government. Some recognize this, some don't. Ultimately, it is the medical staff which has to set the directions. But a lot of it depends upon the administrators; different methods of planning would lead to different ways in which doctors work.

Another physician believes that the ability of the association to achieve its "mission" has been hampered by the degree of competition among some of the hospitals. In addition, this physician maintains that the consortium has not been as successful as it might have because the people who initiated the process of setting it up were administrators rather than physicians. This physician admits:

> Membership in the Consortium has been a good learning experience for me. At this stage I feel much more optimistic with regard to rationalization of the health care system because of the SMHA's presence, and in spite of some blockages, there have been some concrete achievements such as resolution of the CAT scanner issue, a joint pseudo-emergency exercise last year, and an increased sense of awareness among the hospitals of the fiscal constraints on health care.

One member suggests that the association is at a point where they are beginning to coordinate their efforts on less important issues such as collection of bad debts and repair services for biomedical equipment and are also examining whether or not a joint security service could be developed, but that many other management activities such as allocation and regionalization of services are not being seriously addressed.

Others seem to agree with this opinion that the association is in a transitional phase and is slowly moving from the "nuts and bolts to the significant," and they concur that it has been moving too slowly.

> We still are suffering growing up pains. It will take about five years or a little more to achieve the kind of power that the Hartford Consortium has achieved. There is a lot of mistrust among the member hospitals. We are, however, continuously trying to share information and trying to be supportive of each other.

One of the administrators maintains that the consortium has not been successful at all:

> After some initial meetings I realized that they were getting boring and repetitious, that nothing was being accomplished, and that the individuals present were dragging their feet on critical issues. The Consortium has been a failure. It does not have one concrete achievement to show for its existence over two years. All that you witness is a struggle for power between the two giants: Mt. Auburn and Cambridge Hospitals. The Consortium could have organized a central laundry system, a central purchasing system, and a central personnel system. People talk a lot about these things, but nothing ever happens. They never seem to take the discussion to the point where they have to make commitments to change from the established way of doing things. It is all talk, talk, talk. I'm sure that a central purchasing system can help all the hospitals obtain larger discounts on their purchases. But because of politics, the representatives have not done anything to date.

Another member offered this advice:

> I think there are two basic ways in which joint planning can materialize in a multi-institutional system of hospitals. One is eliminating duplication by creating hospitals with different levels of capacity. Thus, there might be one hospital with all the exotic equipment and other services, while all the other hospitals refer to it routinely. The second way is that hospitals sit around a table and divide the pie so that every hospital has some services. There would be no super-hospital with all the services and there would be lots of cross-referrals.

Another administrator stated that he did not know whether or not the association would succeed:

At least Mt. Auburn and Cambridge Hospitals get to talk to each other, and that by itself is a tremendous accomplishment. If you can get the physicians to stop thinking about themselves and their current ideas of what is meant by success, the Consortium might get a big boost.

At the end of five years, one administrator hoped that:

We would have obtained bioengineering needs from one firm, there would be a centralized credit and collection agency, we would have coordinated educational programs for the community, we would have developed more trust among each other as a result of becoming more unified, and the HSA would start regarding the Consortium as a powerful force. We would then be a responsible organization rather than being a rubber stamp only.

Others believe that the association has been low-key and will continue in this vein because there is little economic advantage for the hospitals to do more. Even the federal government has been reluctant to mandate local agencies such as the HSAs to strongly intervene with regular hospital policies.

A physician stated that he felt good about the progress the medical committee has made:

I think that the task forces will definitely make progress over the next few years. There will be progress though it may not be earthshaking. I think the physicians are now quite willing to put forth the time and effort required to make these task forces a success. Also, the Consortium continues to forge ahead, though a little slowly. Barriers of competition are being broken. There is more cooperation and communication. I am more certain of progress in the medical group than in the entire group. What I often think is: how long should we go on accepting the growing pains? Although at this point I feel more optimistic about progress, I also feel that many other consortia have gone much farther ahead than the SMHA.

Another physician recommended that:

The member institutions and the individuals should get to know each other better; each member institution should work at making itself stronger and making the Consortium stronger. We should start with the assumption that the Consortium is going to be effective, and we should accentuate the common achievements.

A recommendation was the possibility of extending membership to Harvard Community Health Plan and the Harvard/M.I.T. Health Services:

> But at this stage we should leave extension at the level of consideration only. Rushing it would emasculate the Association. True, from a long-run point of view, having a membership of just the hospitals is too narrow a base. It is a question of timing and these things should be taken up slowly.

This pessimistic prediction:

> One or another hospital may pull out of the Consortium. In fact, I may be one of those. I think that the issues facing the SMHA are very important and substantive, but the way they are discussed does not lead to productive output.

was followed by an equally optimistic one:

> I think it is a precursor to a conglomerate in the region. When that happens, all we would have to do would be to amend the corporate charter of SMHA. The interim period is mentally preparing the institutions to accept their new role in terms of interinstitutional planning. All the hospitals in this area should be merged. There should be a common policy formation body, one dietary body, one central laboratory, one computer center, and so on. Thus, institution A could be solely for medical care; institution B solely for surgical care; institution C solely for Ob/Gyn, and so on. To maximize economies of scale, one has got to have legislation.

But the more common response regarding the future seems to be summed up in this last comment:

> I really don't know. My involvement in the SMHA is so low that I have given up thinking about it.

Chapter 8

The Capital Area
Health Consortium

In May 1974 eight hospitals in the greater Hartford, Connecticut, area signed the "Hartford Compact," which created the Capital Area Health Consortium. The consortium was created to collectively maintain, improve, and develop a health-care system designed to meet the health needs of the area. The signing of the compact took place in the Old State House, built in 1796, and many who attended considered it to be a historic event.

John Danielson, subsequently the executive director, describes the reasons for its formation:

> It was not put together for purposes of merger which was why most of the large consortiums in this country were put together. The Harvard Consortium was put together as a smoke screen to merge the three cripples; the two Brighams, and the Boston Hospital for Women. The Northwestern Consortium was put together to merge the rehab and the new women's hospital. The Detroit Consortium was put together to combine hospitals to deal largely with the land development problem. The nine hospitals in the Hartford Consortium are all strong, viable, and well managed, and there are no cripples to merge. The agenda was not to develop joint purchasing, or to develop a consortium that would improve management of their hospitals. The hospitals got together for three reasons. One was the former president of Hartford Hospital. You always have to have a Winston Churchill or a Jack Kennedy, or a somebody to make pronouncements and

to visualize and articulate the issues to the people. There he was, a year away from retirement, the dean of the hospitals, an absolutely beautiful human being in every way, and brilliant.

The second reason was that these people had been in touch with what was happening in Washington. Most of them were very active nationally and had anticipated Public Law 93-641, in which four of the ten priorities in health mandated the development of multi-institutional collaboration. They knew that regionalization by some authority was inevitable and that there would be some reorganization of the health care system. They believed that they didn't have to destroy the present system in the process, and if they banded together and structured a consortium that was medically program oriented, i.e., dealing with access, maldistribution, and medical care, rather than "buying brooms better," their group of institutions had the right to self-determination in the public interest.

The right to self-determination has been an inherent entrepreneurial trait of the medical profession for 200 years. There is nothing wrong with being self-serving if it is in the public interest. I think several of our own leaders in medicine have said that the reorganization of the health care system is too important to be left up to doctors. That is nonsense. That is like saying that flying is too important to be left up to pilots. The problem is that in the medical profession we have apologized for what it is that we know how to do better than anyone else.

The third reason was that the physicians instinctively knew that they were now totally dependent upon their hospitals to practice medicine, and that their institutions were their greatest ally and not their greatest adversary. The idea of a self-governing medical staff away from the management and the process of the institution was no longer appealing, and they began to see the self-perpetuating boards of trustees as an inappropriate place for them to have their input.

BACKGROUND

For several years two of Hartford's most prominent physicians had been prodding the Connecticut hospitals to work more closely together. For about twenty years, under one of the doctor's direction, the hospital administrators in the area had met periodically to discuss common issues and problems. At one time a council was formed, only to be abandoned after it was evident that issues could not be resolved within the existing organizational structure of the council.

In late 1972 several events occurred that moved the hospitals in the area closer toward organizing a consortium. The Regional B Planning Agency and the Connecticut Hospital Planning Committee, a voluntary planning group funded mainly by the state's hospitals, urged the hospitals in the Hartford area to make a more strenuous effort to cooperate. Studies of open heart surgery facilities in the city and high-energy radiotherapy facilities in the state had shown duplication and competition for patients. The studies also raised serious questions about the quality of medical care in underused facilities. It was pointed out that the city had several hospitals but no trauma unit and no burn unit, and several other health care needs were not being met. Hartford is the headquarters for some of the nation's largest insurance companies, all of which were expanding their efforts in health insurance. While there was no formal pressure from the companies, they let it be known that the hospitals in the area should work more closely together.

Early in 1973 three representatives from each of the eight hospitals began meeting on a monthly basis to determine if a consortium could be formed. The representatives came from the administration, governing boards, and medical staffs of the hospitals. The University of Connecticut School of Medicine's dean was also named to what became a twenty-five-member steering committee. In spring 1973 the County Medical Society hosted a meeting that included the members of the boards, medical staffs, and executives of all the institutions in the area. At this meeting, unanimous agreement to form a consortium was obtained.

Nevertheless, reactions among the trustees and physicians were varied. Some were enthusiastic, some were dubious, and none seemed to know how to accomplish the task of developing a consortium. They believed that their biggest problem would be to obtain approval from their respective medical staffs. In one hospital the board of trustees ordered the physicians to get involved. In another, the administrators explained the advantages and disadvantages to the physicians, and the trustees asked them to join in. For the most part, the administrators carried the message to the medical staffs. Each hospital was left to its own devices to obtain the physician's support. The major questions that physicians had tended to ask revolved around common medical staff privileges: Would there be an adequate match if a physician from one hospital made use of facilities at another hospital, and would physicians, particularly surgeons from hospital A, fill up beds and operating time at hospital B?

A number of issues were initially agreed on to resolve many preliminary conflicts. It was decided that staff privileges at all the hospitals would not just be bestowed on all the physicians in the area. A physician interested in access to another hospital would have to make a request for privileges to that particular hospital, and acceptance or rejection of such a request would be determined by the affected hospital. It was also agreed that the board of trustees of each of the hospitals could not be denied the right to appoint any three members they chose to the consortium board.

The physicians organized themselves into a committee and began to work on writing up a set of consortium bylaws. The bylaws were approved in March 1974, and they state that the purpose of the consortium is to coordinate and further the health care delivery, medical, educational, research, administrative, and other activities of its members in order to provide:

a. the highest possible quality of medical services at the lowest practicable cost to all people needing such services
b. the most advanced coordinated programs possible in the areas of preventive care and research
c. the coordination of members' service to eliminate to the greatest possible degree both unnecessary duplication and incomplete coverage in the providing of services and facilities
d. the greatest possible integration of educational programs in medicine, dentistry, nursing, and allied health
e. the education of the public as to the health-care needs of the community and the goals of the corporation.

A board of trustees was established and consisted of a trustee, physician, and administrative representative from each of the hospitals. The University of Connecticut Health Center was permitted a fourth member, the dean of its medical school. This was done because one of the fundamental foundations of the consortium was that the medical school, being new in Connecticut, was a "hospital without walls," and used the clinical environment of the consortium hospitals for its first four classes, which produced an element of educational value that tied all the hospitals together. In addition, the new medical school produced the reversal of the usual "town-gown" situation because the medical school was more dependent on the hospitals than they were on the medical school. John Danielson was chosen to be the executive director of the consortium and became an ex officio member of the board.

The power of the consortium is contained in a section of the bylaws that covers rights and obligations. There is a dollar limit on the cost of a capital improvement that can be made without approval of the trustees. There are also obligations in the areas of budgets and financial statements, sharing of services and facilities, common standards of care, and a pledge to cooperate with one another. A specific power given to the board is "to monitor the quality of patient care provided by its members, to prescribe standards of patient care with specific reference to preventive care and inpatient and outpatient care, and alone or in cooperation with others to implement programs designed to attain and maintain the highest standards possible among its members in all areas of patient care." After ninety days' notice, any member can resign. If the trustees vote in the majority, any nonprofit hospital in the Capital Area may join.

All the hospitals in the greater Hartford area participated in the formation of the consortium with the exception of Veterans' Administration Hospital, which could not then join for two reasons: (1) the federal government cannot delegate or abdicate its responsibility for determining its resources to a private corporation, and (2) the federal government cannot be assessed by any private corporation, and it had been written into the original set of bylaws that "assessment of its members" would take place.

The Veterans' Administration Hospital did eventually join the consortium in May 1975 because the members decided to use consensus to decide new programs and resource allocation, which allowed the federal hospital and also the state hospital (University of Connecticut School of Medicine-John Dempsey Hospital) to become bonafide members. The hospital arrangement was formalized in November 1975.

The hospitals vary in size and have different strengths and abilities. They comprise about 30 percent of Connecticut's total hospital beds, and provide services and facilities to an estimated 1.5 million people. They include about 2500 physicians and dentists, who represent approximately 40 percent of the total of those professionals in the state. The participating hospitals include the University of Connecticut-John Dempsey Hospital, School of Medicine, and Veterans' Administration Hospital; St. Francis Hospital; Newington Children's Hospital; New Britain General Hospital; Mt. Sinai Hospital; Manchester Memorial Hospital; The Institute of Living; and Hartford Hospital.

ORGANIZATION AND MANAGEMENT

The first six months after the consortium was established were devoted to developing an appropriate organizational structure. A great deal of effort went into this, as it was considered to be fundamental to everything that was to follow. A considerable amount of time during this period was also spent by the executive director, John Danielson, in developing an in-depth understanding of the member institutions since they were considered to be very different from one another. An area of major concern and activity in the early stages of the consortium was to develop good working relationships with the other health care delivery resources in the area.

Several critical questions were raised by the hospitals when they addressed the issue of sharing services:

Who pays for the transportation when a patient from one hospital must be taken by ambulance to the hospital that is housing a particular diagnostic tool (e.g., CAT scanner)?

Who has the legal responsibility for the patient in the case of malpractice?

Who does the billing for the service and under what auspices?

Do the consortium hospitals regard themselves as partners or consumers of one another?

Should the consortium develop a patient information system and common medical records that would allow the members to give themselves a continuing evaluation of their performance?

A medical staff committee was formed, with its first task being to develop a set of medical staff bylaws. They dealt with three key issues.

They decided that every doctor who was going to be involved had to have a primary appointment and be on the active staff of one of the member hospitals. Second, they decided that if a physician had a primary appointment at one of the member hospitals, the other hospitals would regard the credentials committee of the primary hospital as being equal to theirs in judgment. Third, they decided that whatever staff a physician went on to admit a patient, he would have to follow that hospital's rules and regulations and bylaws, not those from his primary hospital. The members felt that this would protect the integrity, sovereignty, and individuality of every medical staff.

Concurrent with the development of the medical committee, an administrative committee was appointed, and its members were given the task of setting standards for the operation of the consortium. One of their greatest fears was that they were going to lose their "walls" and become a kind of a "potpourri." They wanted to avoid making every hospital the same. The members decided in the very beginning that they would regard each hospital as separate. They felt it was important to regard each other as different and wanted to protect the sovereignty of each institution.

Danielson commented:

If you put people who are different around a table, you can get to the issue of consensus because they can regard each other as being of equal competence. It is then not difficult to bring them to the same goals and objectives.

The second issue that the administrative committee decided on was that the last thing they needed was an insecure institution and that the financial and service viability of every institution was essential. The committee members felt that the consortium should not do anything that would render any member hospital insecure because insecure institutions, like insecure people, don't give, and the issue fundamental to the consortium was sharing. The members were convinced that the strength of the consortium was going to be in the strength of its individual members. They decided that it would be in their best interest to help each other rather than to carve each other up. The consortium was not to be a merger, a holding company, a mini hospital association, a hospital system with one dominant institution controlling, or a joint purchasing and/or management council. It was something new: a health consortium whose members had the same value judgments and agreed on the same goals and objectives.

After writing and signing the charter and bylaws and hiring an executive director, the next task was to establish a philosophy of how the consortium was to be managed and an acceptable decision-making process. Since the goals and objectives were already stated in the charter and bylaws, the decision-making process and an appropriate organizational structure were of the highest priority.

An ad hoc committee was appointed to address this task. The committee decided that:

The consortium would seek to protect each member's integrity and sovereignty. The consortium should be a mosaic made up of a variety of separate entities that retain their characters, colors, and identities and when put together represent a "new" identity capable of accomplishing what each could not do alone.

The consortium need not cripple one member by sacrificing its strengths to favor the weaknesses of another and that duplication (not redundancy) may be in the public interest in order to improve access to care and that the removal of a critical service could destroy the viability of the institution.

The strength of the consortium rests in the strengths of its members, and this is truly in the public interest.

John Danielson suggested to the members that they use the method of voting when deciding on matters of "process," that is, voting on the bylaws, minutes of meetings, committee membership, organization, and structure. However, he advised them to use consensus when dealing with "outcome oriented" activities because he felt that none of the member hospitals would be willing to discuss anything really worthwhile if they were forced to vote on matters that affected their institutional viability, that is, resource and program allocation. It is relatively easy to obtain a consensus if there is no serious conflict of interest between the institutions, if there are no serious financial implications, or if the status of the individual institutions is not threatened. If the members of the group had difficulty in reaching a consensus, Danielson said that it was his responsibility and the responsibility of all the members to work toward the resolution of the conflict.

The committee agreed that:

If they were to regard each other as being of equal competence and of having the capability of contributing some special expertise in their specific area of consortium participation, the decision-making process could not be by vote but needed to be by consensus.

Since there would be occasions when there was insufficient time to convene the members but action was required, each institution had the right to act independently with this understanding—that consensus would be sought retrospectively. However, if consensus were deemed impossible, a vote would be taken.

There would be four councils reporting to the board of trustees (see Figure 8.1). Each of these councils has advisory committees that represent the specialization and unique competence within the hospitals to which the councils may refer any matter for expert advice.

Professional Staff Council: medicine, pediatrics, obstetrics/gynecology, psychiatry, pathology and laboratory, radiology, nursing, ambulatory care, dentistry, anesthesiology, and malpractice.

Mangement Council: medical libraries, medical records, finance, information and data exchange, medical social services, personnel, and purchasing agents.

Council on Education and Research: allied health, graduate medical education, patient education. Some twenty-two standing committees with five ad hoc committees now meet.

Hospital Trustees Council: composed of the trustees from each of the hospitals.

The consortium staff would remain small and consist of an executive director, administrative assistant (office manager), and clerical assistance. In order to accomplish this goal, the members

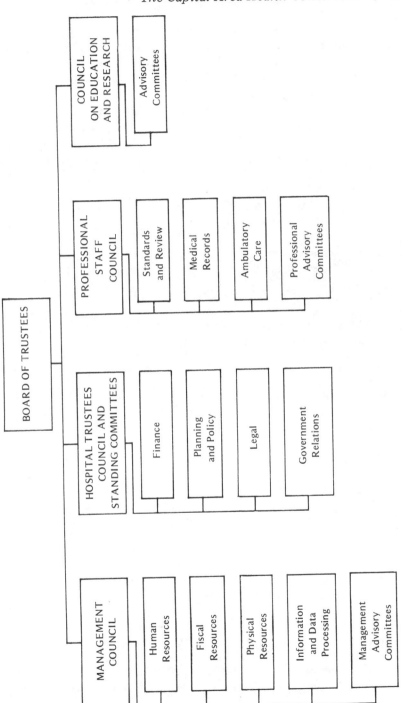

Figure 8.1. Organization Chart: Capital Area Health Consortium, Inc.

agreed that the executive director could enlist the talent existing within the member institutions to work on consortium projects and that by and large the hospitals would operate the various essential programs with some initiation and coordination by the consortium office.

There should be a clear-cut role established for the executive director.

Executive Director: Responsibilities and Skills

On February 7, 1975, the goals and objectives committee approved the following role of the executive director:

> He should be the chief executive officer of the Corporation responsible to the board of trustees for the management and general supervision of its activities and staff.
>
> The executive director shall act on behalf of the Consortium only when he is certain that a consensus has been reached or a vote taken. He should make himself available as a consultant to the member hospitals upon request. He should be encouraged to give advice and counsel to legislative and government representatives, but to abstain from the role of lobbyist. He should represent the interests of not only the member hospitals, but of the public as well, and only when these are determined to be compatible. He should facilitate the clarification of the public needs for health care. He should be the spokesman for the value of the programs that improve the "quality of life" and the productivity of the citizens which are often obscured by the addiction to measuring all worth in terms of cost-per-unit service.
>
> On the other hand, he should not represent the individual hospitals regarding the effectiveness of their own fiscal affairs. With as complete knowledge as it is possible of each hospital, its program and its needs, he should act as a catalyst in developing understanding and consensus among them as well as' coordinating their efforts. His personal conduct should be such as to reflect favorably upon the member institutions.

John Danielson has explicitly tried to create an atmosphere of trust among the consortium members.

> We approach problems so that no one is going to be badly hurt. If somebody is bleeding we all go to help that person rather than to encourage the basic human animal instinct to kill a bleeding and wounded tiger. You don't need a wounded tiger in the bush. You either kill him or cure him, but don't leave him there. We try to help somebody who is in

trouble because someone in trouble is going to be a problem and a real difficulty to the system. And it is my job to try and convince them of that and to keep them talking together. It is an extraordinarily difficult thing to do.

The greatest problems usually arise among the group of administrators rather than the physicians. According to John Danielson:

It is with the administrators where the greatest conflict occurs because it is they who have always seen the reward system in terms of those things that they can control; not those things that they cannot control. They are very unsophisticated when it comes to managing patients; however, they are extraordinarily sophisticated when it comes to managing things.

John Danielson functions as a personal consultant. He knows the members personally and therefore they trust him to interpret for them when something is going wrong, and can steer them back to the right track. But most of all, he keeps them from killing each other.

Most hospital administrators do not understand that the real issue is the management of patient care and that is why I am involved in what I am doing here. The issue is the management of patient care. It is not the management of things. I view the institutions as if they were biological entities. They ingest, digest, excrete, throw up, get sick, have personalities, get nervous, they are suspicious, they are competitive, they are everything. Each institution is a biological entity; it has a clear characteristic personality and what it does is never accidental. It has always got a reason. It is my job to know what that reason is. It is the same with people, so I regard them as people. I do not see 3,800 beds in front of me at the board meetings, I see nine people.

If the institutions were put together the way they are in Chicago, New York, Detroit, or Los Angeles, the circumstances would be different, and they would do things differently. What they have done is taken a set of circumstances with their given resources and developed a structure that is right for them. It is not transferable. John Danielson divides his attention and efforts into four categories: those things that are functional and amenable to change, those things that are dysfunctional and amenable to change, those things that are dysfunctional and not possible to change, and those things that are functional but not possible to change. Since situations are never static but often shift from one category to another, it is important in his role as executive director to be aware of all the possibilities. He describes his role as executive director as follows:

My job is neither to control the members personally or to run their affairs, but is to be able to put those tigers on the stools so the act will be performed, and when a tiger is off the stool, I have got to find him and get him back on the stool, or the people will want their money back. I do not jump through the hoops and I do not do the performance. All I am in there for is to make sure that everybody else does their thing successfully so we all come out of it okay.

He sees himself as a "facilitator." He is the person who helps the group know when they have reached a consensus.

We can get consensus prospectively or we can get consensus retrospectively. It does not make any difference. If we get consensus retrospectively, what we have done is a beautiful thing. It tells everybody what we did and why. Now if we were wrong and could not get consensus retrospectively, we would all agree to help figure out some way to deal with what had been done. Everybody is going to make mistakes. All we have to agree to is to put the issue on the table. We start talking about it and agree that no one will act until the group has been brought to a consensus. That is my job.

There are two times when the consensus approach will not work. One is when there is not enough time. The consortium was never meant to constipate the institutions and be another authority. It was meant to be a facilitator and was supposed to make their job easier, quicker, and better so that they could be in charge of their own strategy, and could take the intent of Congress and meet it, but bend the regulations. No one would ever hold them to be irresponsible if they bent the regulations but fulfilled the intent of Congress.

The second time the consensus approach will not work is if the consortium has 50 percent of the cards, and the federal government or the HSA or somebody in authority holds the other hand. If you are told that you can have only one cardiac surgery program in Hartford, since both St. Francis Hospital and Hartford Hospital have cardiac surgery programs, talking for a thousand years would never result in consensus.

What happened in this situation is that they began to review the options:

That is my job, to help those two institutions come up with alternatives. It is very important not to just accept what somebody says, but to examine the reasons why there only ought to be one cardiac surgery program in Hartford. After quite a bit of deliberation, they decided to keep both heart surgery programs, since the capital investment was already there, and move the team instead of the people. Why move the patients if you can move the team? They joined the two heart surgery teams together into one and began to operate in both places.

He admits that the members came up with that alternative:

> With a little help. Somebody has got to help them. There has always got to be somebody around to help them.

He believes that an executive director should not be hired for a consortium board until the "process" has been decided. Once this has occurred, he suggests, the implementation of the process should become the job of the executive director. He suggests that there are four loyalties that are constant companions to the board members:

> First is the loyalty to their own hospital. Second is the loyalty to the profession that they represent, or their ethic and its effort. The third is the loyalty to the patient and to the community. The fourth is the loyalty to the Consortium. It is my job to make sure that the loyalty to this Consortium is not in conflict with the other three.

One of the most difficult things he has had to contend with is keeping a "low profile" and getting the members to understand that the consortium is theirs, not his.

For those who are interested in becoming an executive director of a consortium, he gives the following advice:

> Somebody once asked me what kind of textbook I would recommend for reading material, and I said, "there is only one and that is the Bible." Read the Bible and you will know how to run a consortium. It is all there.

ACCOMPLISHMENTS

While views vary as to whether the consortium has made a significant difference to what might have been done anyway, there are a number of examples of programs and projects that the consortium has developed through a joint and cooperative effort among its members.

Community Cancer Control Program. The consortium signed a subcontract with the State Department of Health that had applied for a National Cancer Institute Community Cancer Control Planning grant in order to establish a public/private partnership in planning for the implementation of a comprehensive intervention for three sites of cancer—breast, colon, and lung. The most important part of this contractual agreement was to demonstrate by example the need for public/private partnership on the basis that when one or the other failed to meet its obligation, the other participant would lend its support and effort to make the project a success. Although it was not anticipated that it would be required to meet this responsibility so soon, the death of the principal investigator for the statewide project and severe financial constraints on the State Department of Health made it imperative that the consortium take on a temporary leadership role. The consortium responded and reorganized the project with the help of the Health Department and the State Cancer Consortium. The project was moved to the University of Connecticut Health Center. The consortium facilitated the hiring of a new principal investigator and a project director, and reallocated the resources. In a period of three weeks, the National Cancer Institute signed on to the new agreement and gave immediate recognition that the public/private partnership had worked in the interest of the people of the state of Connecticut.

Nursing Project. A very special and unique project in nursing has been developed and submitted to the Kellogg Foundation for consideration. This project would use the methodology established by Conedics of Johnson & Johnson to examine, in a nonjudgmental way, all the positions in nursing services, establishing current expectations of those positions, and testing the competence of the individual employees holding those positions. They would validate the description of the nursing process by individual nursing stations and develop a tool to test for competency that would be used in the hiring of any nursing personnel for these positions. The impact of this would be to identify an orientation and on-the-job training program directed specifically to the individual applicant's needs, thus saving thousands of hours of unnecessary training. It would further provide an opportunity for consortium-wide recruiting and orientation programs that could have savings to the consortium hospitals of hundreds of thousands of dollars. The project also would have a concurrent project for measuring patient outcomes based on criteria established in a program of quality assurance and nursing audit that is currently in process at various institutions. It is intended to bring the nursing process as determined by Conedics and patient outcomes based on established criteria together at the end of a three-year period, thereby identifying clearly the priorities in nursing practice that affect patient outcome and the elimination and/or addition to that practice as measured by results. This would ultimately place in the hands of the consortium nursing departments a presently non-existent tool that would prove the worth of the practice of nursing and the potential of actually charging patients for services rendered.

Rehabilitation. The consortium staff has been working with the Newington Children's Hospital and the various councils to establish a consortium-wide program for rehabilitation for children and adults. A plan was proposed to establish an adult unit at Newington Children's Hospital with the understanding that none of the other member hospitals would establish major rehabilitation programs including the University of Connecticut Health Center. Assurances through the consortium councils have been given by all participating members that the focus of the consortium rehabilitation program would be located at Newington Children's Hospital and that a cooperative relationship would be developed in order to provide a major comprehensive and coordinated program in rehabilitation that would include the support and participation of the private health agencies within the community as well. The consortium is currently developing a strategy for the presentation of this program to the Commission on Hospitals and Health Care with the intent of obtaining an approval for a Certificate of Need.

Regional Neonatology Program. A regional neonatology program hasbeen organized by the consortium pediatric advisory committee of the professional staff council that provides for various levels of care for the newborn, utilizing the resources of the involved institutions. This program is coordinated and directed from the department of pediatrics at the University of Connecticut Health Center.

Consortium-Affiliated Medical and Dental Staff. In order to provide the most efficient and effective system that would facilitate access by the public to any and all of the available resources, a vehicle was needed to ensure proper distribution of manpower and facilities, as well as a method of considering the consolidation and coordination of medical services to avoid unnecessary duplication. This was accomplished by the development of a set of bylaws governing consortium-wide access to medical staff membership by any physician who held a primary staff appointment in one of the consortium hospitals.

Alcohol Program. Although six of the members founded the Combined Hospitals Alcohol Program before the existence of the consortium, there has been a continuous effort on the part of the consortium staff to help in the reorganization and ultimate success of this medical program.

Graduate Medical Education. A major effort is currently underway to develop a unified program in graduate medical education for the consortium hospitals. A special committee has presented its first draft to the Council on Education and Research, and there is every indication that the Capital Area Health Consortium will establish a model in the development of university-connected programs in graduate medical education. It is hoped that by such initiative it will be able to influence the regulation of federal legislation in this area.

Patient Education. A major effort has been made to establish a consortium-wide program for patient education that would be hospital based. Connecticut Blue Cross has pledged $20,000 to the hiring of a coordinator for such a program, and a representative committee is at work developing this effort.

Allied Health. One of the most important efforts in consolidating education programs is currently under consideration by the University of Connecticut and the Consortium Committee on Allied Health. The proposal has been made that all clinical experience for the students of the Schools of Allied Health at the University of Connecticut be concentrated in the consortium hospitals and that once this program is approved and implemented, the university will be in a position to move its School of Allied Health to the Hartford area as has been mandated by the board of regents.

Consortium Medical Librarians. One of the most effective programs in sharing thus far developed has been the Capital Area Health Consortium's librarian's program. Significant cost savings have been experienced to date through the assignment to a specific hospital of the consortium the responsibility of purchasing and sharing certain journals most applicable to their expertise. Through this accomplishment the consortium has essentially a single medical library for consortium hospitals. The current problem is to develop efficient and effective means of transporting the material between hospitals. A major document has been printed showing the location of all such shared periodicals, journals, and textbooks.

Nurse Training Oncology Workshop. A workshop for the training of nurse specialists in oncology was developed under the consortium auspices with the cooperation of the Visiting Nurse Association.

Open Heart Surgery. This program is essentially confined to two participating hospitals, Hartford Hospital and St. Francis Hospital. The cooperation between these two institutions has resulted in the sharing of facilities, equipment, and manpower.

The consortium developed a position on its responsibility for care of the elderly including long-term beds.

The consortium monitored, facilitated, and negotiated the budget process with the Commission on Hospitals and Health Care and is in the process of developing a procedure for handling the review of all major capital equipment and programs.

The consortium took a strong position in opposition to the approval of a proprietary, freestanding ambulatory care center in Hartford; and through consortium efforts, managed to have their position sustained by the Commission on Hospitals and Health Care. It is in the process of developing a consortium-wide review and commitment to ambulatory surgery centers that are part of the hospital delivery system.

It had been actively involved with the staff of the Health Planning Council in the development of an HSA within its region in order to not only influence the regulations to be written, but to initiate necessary changes that the members believe reflect the intent of Congress for Public Law 93-641.

Evaluation and the Future

Never one to be satisfied, John Danielson reminded the consortium board in July 1976 of their early concerns and suggested that they review where they were and whether their fears and hopes had come true.

A special retreat meeting of the consortium's board of trustees was held in October 1976. Its purpose was to reexamine their original strategy, programs, and assumptions in light of what appeared to be an identity crisis spawned out of overexpectations and perceived underachievement during the consortium's first two years of operation. The president suggested that they establish a new strategy if necessary and agree on the appropriate tactics to accomplish their goals and objectives. He asked the following questions:

Has the Commission on Hospitals and Health Care created a new and different "ball game"? Do we want to become an "arm" of the Commission—must we be this in order to establish credibility? Have we forgotten our long-term objectives? What is our role in this new environment where economics seem to be the sole judge of quality?

It was established that the consortium was indeed unique. Consequently, there were no other models for them to examine or learn from. They decided to evaluate the outcome of their five original concerns and came to the following conclusions:

Concern: That strong, viable, and independent hospitals would become subject to the authority of the consortium, thus sacrificing their institutional integrity and identity.

Conclusion: This had not happened. As a matter of fact, they may have been too successful in solving this concern by spending an inordinate amount of time and effort in "keeping the peace," and helping to solve individual institutional problems.

Concern: That there would be a lack of responsiveness and that this would be another authority to complicate the decision-making process.

Conclusion: This did not occur since the consortium by its very presence is a restraining force, and those issues requiring consideration and consensus were reasonable and easily agreed to.

Concern: That the consortium would threaten the financial viability of its members through the crippling effect of dividing and concentrating services and facilities.

Conclusion: To date, no hospital had been injured by any premature or capricious decision that would eliminate necessary services. They were not overbedded or irresponsibly planned, but it was pointed out that unless they were vigilant, they could be coerced into becoming an arm of the commission, leaving no organizational structure to protect the public's right to full access and quality care.

Concern: That the consortium would be able to justify through money savings the contributions of its members.

Conclusion: This had been a serious question raised by the members themselves that the consortium may be criticized for its lack of accomplishment in cutting costs and services. It was at this point that emphasis was made in support of the consortium as one representative of the hospitals' concern for the health needs of the community, the quality of care, ample access to the services, and the many programs that deal with health maintenance and quality of life. It was suggested that the consortium must be that countervalent force that meets the intense new thrust of the commission to control health care by controlling price and volume. It was agreed that the consortium did not and should not accept "adequate care" whenever that is defined to mean less care by fewer people for less money at less quality.

Concern: That the undertaking was too ambitious and would lead to overexpectations.

Conclusion: To some extent this was true and might have been the seed of their frustration with limited, tangible accomplishments in the short period of time the consortium had been in operation.

Several tactics utilized by the consortium were also reviewed, and the assumptions regarding them were examined:

Tactic: The decision-making process was to be by consensus, using the same rules that govern vote.

Conclusion: This system had worked well to date, even though at times consensus was thought to be achieved when in fact it had not been. It was pointed out that this was a necessary procedure in order to retain the University Medical Center and the Veterans' Administration Hospital as members. The important consideration was whether the basis of the trust upon which they built the consortium was worthy of their belief and commitment.

Tactic: Consortium identity is dependent on sharing credit for what the members do.

Conclusion: Although the hospitals could identify their relationship to the consortium by letterhead, sign, and/or acknowledgment, it was determined that the consortium must develop its own identifiable programs and serve its members in a more tangible way.

Tactic: Consortium staff would remain small, and the necessary expertise required to initiate and study consortium-wide programs would come on loan from the member institutions.

Conclusion: This was unrealistic since the pressure of the members' primary responsibility to their hospitals had increased, leaving little or no time for consortium activities. It was pointed out that the resources of the institutions were under attack and community-wide health programs could be a serious distraction of time and money. It was decided that separate short-term staffing would be contracted for each of the major program developments, including consultation advice.

Tactic: By their collective effort and unified approach in combining their resources, they would cause the Commission on Hospitals and Health Care to treat their members differently in review of budgets and consideration of their requests.

Conclusion: This did not happen. The Commission on Hospitals and Health Care virtually ignored the presence of the consortium, even though the executive director spoke at several of the budget hearings. Some new strategy needed to be developed in order for the consortium to have a significant impact on the commission in its deliberations.

A new strategy was developed. The consortium would be program oriented in its next phase of development, which they hoped would solve several of the critical problems confronting them:

a. The consortium would have identity through its new program planning.
b. The staff would be augmented by expert, paid consultants and advisors.
c. The consortium would seek outside funding for these projects, but not for their implementations. The hospitals, through commission pass-through of cost or through other third-party payer, would finance the implementation.
d. Through total and comprehensive program planning, they would be able to present a consortium plan before the commission rather than an individual hospital request. If the hospital request was a part of an overall plan, the commission would be required to view the request as a significant and critical part of a health plan for the people of the greater Hartford area. It was hoped that this would begin to force the commission to recognize the consortium in a different light.
e. It was further decided that the board of trustees of the consortium would meet monthly and that the president and the executive director would from time to time invite visitors who had particular concerns and expertise regarding the health field to meet with them, for example, HSA, health department people, legislative representatives, Blue Cross representatives, and representatives from other insurance companies.

The Views of Some Principal Participants

A former president of Hartford Hospital, of the American Hospital Association, and of the Capital Area Health Consortium is credited as being the originator of the consortium. He retired in 1976 from his position at Hartford Hospital and assumed the position of acting director of the John Dempsey Hospital-University of Connecticut Medical School until a permanent director was appointed.

He had received the highest respect and trust from the health professionals in the Hartford area as well as nationwide for several years. His work toward the formation of a consortium was considered by many to be his last "statesman-like effort" before he retired from Hartford Hospital, rather than a scheme on his part to increase his or Hartford Hospital's power.

This physician's greatest hope is that the consortium achieve enough cooperation among the member hospitals for it to become more of a system. He hopes that eventually St. Francis Hospital can become a center for high-risk pregnancies, Hartford Hospital for kidney transplants, the Health Center for neonatology, and the Newington Children's Hospital for rehabilitation. The public must be made to understand that in areas such as general surgery, medicine and obstetrics, the Capital Area is large enough to support multiple facilities. In terms of obstetric cases especially, the units in St. Francis, Hartford, and Mt. Sinai are big enough to be practical as well as cost effective.

A chief of staff of one of the hospitals on the board remembers that when the ideas about starting up a consortium were first circulated, the responses of the physicians were quite varied. Some of them were less than enthusiastic, although not totally hostile. But the founder had the ability of commanding respect from virtually every group he dealt with, and everyone listened to him because they assumed his ideas must have merit. He demonstrated institutional humility, something that was appreciated by the other institutions, who knew that Hartford Hospital was the biggest and the best.

The movement to form the consortium, he said, came from the hospital administrators. From their standpoint it was a way to buffer themselves against tremendous external pressures. It made more sense to them to try to get together than remain separate because the Hospital Cost Commission was coming along, and the wage and price controls were on the horizon.

One of the perceived advantages of the consortium was that it would limit the power of the new medical school. The private sector is always afraid that the university is going to come in and take over, and many doctors were worried that the university physicians were going to take over all their patients and tell them how to practice medicine. If they had a consortium, then they could at least talk to each other, and if the university got too preemptive and too strong, they would be able to hold them in check.

However, the hospital trustees have been very removed from the realities of what goes on in the hospital, and the chief of staff believes that there has to be more intimate involvement by the trustees in the whole process.

His roles on the professional staff council and the board are twofold. One was the responsibility to feed into the consortium the concerns of his medical staff, and the other was to feed back to his medical staff an account of the activities of what was going on at the consortium level.

The biggest advantage of the consortium has been simply sitting down in a room and working together with other health professionals. The physicians turned out to have been the most responsive and responsible group within the consortium in terms of really working together. The least responsive group, in his view, have been the hospital administrators. But most of the physicians do not know what the consortium is all about and what it has been doing. The consortium has not been around long enough, and there have not been enough visible and significant happenings to get the average physician involved. Nevertheless, early involvement of key physicians was important because the consortium could not function without them, and they can be persuasive with their colleagues.

One trustee of Hartford Hospital was an early participant in the consortium's formation, and the founder first discussed his ideas with him as far back as 1971. He and others went along out of respect for his national reputation.

While the major purpose of the consortium was to develop regional coordination of the health care delivery system in the Hartford Capital area, one of the most difficult tasks for Hartford Hospital has been to recognize its responsibility to aid the other participating hospitals.

This trustee feels that the major role of the hospital trustee is to support the consortium, not only at the consortium meetings but at their home institutions as well. On several occasions issues would come up at meetings at Hartford Hospital in the executive committee or the joint conference committee, and participants would have to be reminded by the trustees, "shouldn't this go through the consortium?" A hospital trustee must not be so identified with the daily operations of his own institution that he is likely to forget about the consortium, and he should not let others forget either.

One of the benefits of the consortium is that everyone goes to meetings and talks about problems that they wouldn't ordinarily talk about, and fears seem to dissipate just from this. The consortium is a type of forum where problems are brought up and discussed and "people just can't get up and walk out." One of John Danielson's masterful techniques has been to keep people talking, and sooner or later a solution seems to evolve if people talk with each other long enough.

Danielson was the unanimous choice of the search committee from among numerous applicants. But he is skeptical of the long-term benefits of the consortium because he believes that institutions have tremendous inertia and resistance to giving up anything to anybody else. Physicians are content with their own little practices and do not like change. The St. Francis reluctance he attributes to long-standing competitiveness between hospitals of different religious persuasions. In the future the hospitals will have to place more emphasis on determining priorities:

> If we don't exercise good management techniques and we don't involve everybody in the planning and establishing of priorities, we could have a mess on our hands. But I like to believe that we have the kind of management, medical staff, and trustee involvement which will enable us to muddle our way through without any catastrophies.

An administrator at New Britain General Hospital agrees that one of the basic achievements the consortium has brought about has been the facilitation of communication between colleagues. The three members who belong to the consortium from each hospital have begun to recognize that they not only have a responsibility to their own hospital but to the consortium as well, and in the long run, especially as they get pinched economically, the hospitals will begin to see a need to change hospital programs to consortium programs.

Administrators, unlike physicians who are very independent and don't like teams, have a tendency to be extroverts and are willing to work on committees and teams and listen to many inputs because they have learned that helps them be successful.

Another trustee, from St. Francis Hospital, sees three major achievements. The first is that they now have common medical staff bylaws for all the hospitals. The second is that there has been an increased awareness among the different hospital representatives of each other's problems, and the third is that the trustees, the administrators, and the physicians are now very aware of what makes a hospital work.

One of the major bottlenecks was in getting the physicians involved in the consortium. He suggests that there are two kinds of physicians: the hospital-based physicians and private attendings. The hospital-based physicians readily accepted the consortium philosophy while the attending physicians did not.

He discussed the issue of the consortium with the physicians at St. Francis Hospital. He told them it was essential that they get together with their colleagues from the other hospitals, as well as with the administrators and the trustees from the other hospitals. He stressed that it was about time that each institution stopped looking within and started looking without.

The president of the consortium runs the board meetings. He attends a few meetings of the administrative staff and the professional council. He still regards the first president, from whom he took over in February 1976, as the "godfather" of the consortium. The first president represented the administrators, and the second president represents the trustees. He expects that the third president will be a physician and that the position will keep rotating among the three disciplines. Two other leaders of the consortium have also left, and consequently the consortium is going through a leadership change.

An administrator from St. Francis Hospital does not feel that the consortium has accomplished a great deal. Many of the issues dealt with in the consortium could have been worked out successfully even without the consortium because the administrators among the various hospitals have always had a good relationship with one another. Admitting that the hospitals have been competitive, this administrator thinks they have still tried to cooperate with one another. He was responsible for a change in the bylaws to stipulate that no hospital be required to give up an existing service. He feared that St. Francis Hospital's radiation service would be swallowed up by Hartford Hospital, which at the time was constructing a large radiation center.

This administrator approves of the manner in which the open heart surgery issue was handled by the consortium:

> We have had open heart surgery here for a number of years, but frankly, we had a very poor program. We never got it off the ground and Hartford Hospital had a very successful program. The Commission wanted us to give up our program, but we were reluctant to do so. About two years ago, the surgeons from Hartford Hospital approached us and asked if they could do

heart surgery here because Hartford Hospital had really reached its capacity. At that point in time we were generating about 75 to 80 cases a year through our catherization lab, but the patients were all going to Boston or New York for their surgery. The Hartford Hospital surgeons approached us and asked if they could use our facility, and we of course agreed. Once they came here, we started to increase the number of cases done here, because the referrals started to go to them rather than to Boston. The reason the referrals went to Boston was that the private practitioners felt if they sent their patients to Hartford Hospital they would lose their patients.

They had a public hearing for us. John Danielson wanted us to present it as a joint program, but I was opposed to that because it is not a joint program. We have our facility; we have our nurses. The only thing we share, really are the surgeons. Because they are independent contractors, they do not belong to Hartford Hospital nor to St. Francis Hospital. So we went in as two hospitals with two programs. Hartford Hospital helped us a great deal by stating that they just could not handle the load and they did not wish to handle all the heart cases because they did not want to be identified as the cardiovascular hospital because this would have had an effect on the other types of surgery, and if they devoted too many of their resources to open heart surgery, they would certainly lose general surgery.

One of the problems confronting the consortium is the time frame in which issues are brought up at the various staff committee and board meetings:

We might be talking about things for six months at St. Francis and it might leak out. You have to get all of the proper approvals and commitments at your own institution and find out if it is financially feasible, so you don't really know when to approach it at the Consortium level because there is the danger if you open up too soon, other people latch on to the idea; might have greater resources and might beat you to it. I think it is extremely frustrating for John Danielson. This has come up several times in the past when he felt that he really had not been dealt with properly.

St Francis's administrator is critical of the consortium's executive director:

Our executive director really has not been out on the forefront. I think he should have a high profile. I've done a lot of lobbying myself. I have friends in the legislature. I really do not think it is my job. I think every little bit helps, but I think he should be out there fighting for the hospitals. In fact, the first year he didn't even attend a budget meeting. This was the Commission on Hospitals and Health Care and it was a tough Commission. John Danielson says he really didn't feel it was necessary that he be there because he couldn't really respond to any questions on a particular budget since he had just recently accepted the position of executive director. My idea of a director is to be a person that is going to get out there to know the people, get to know the legislators, get to know the people in the State Department of Health. Now he has a lot to do with the people in the Department of Health. I do not know how much influence he has. I think he is doing it but in a different way than I would do it. So I think it is probably our style. He, for instance, reaches all decisions by a consensus approach. I don't know whether you can do this, whether it is possible, because ultimately, there has to be someone that says, "this is the way it is going to be," at the state level or a higher level. But I do not know whether we could handle that, frankly, in this Consortium; so maybe consensus is the best thing. I had just expected someone that was more visible and better known. Maybe my expectations are too high. John Danielson, I think, has the feeling that he has to be visible on the national scene. I maintain, what good is that doing me? You know, sure, if he wants to go to Washington and pick up some of the news from Washington, fine. But to go around talking about the Consortium, I do not think that does me any good at all. We are not trying to sell the Consortium now. We have it because we want to do something for the Hartford hospitals.

This administrator concedes that John Danielson is in a difficult position:

As he said one day, "you people have something to go home to—I don't." We each have our own hospital. We sit in a group but we know we're going back to run something. He really has nothing because he is sort of under our command, and so it must be a rather frustrating position to be in.

He believes that most doctors do not really want to work at more than one hospital. Some of his doctors go to Mt. Sinai Hospital, but only because it is a five-minute drive from St. Francis. Physicians find it too difficult, and it takes too much out of them, although in fact some of the physicians at St. Francis have applied for staff privileges at some of the other hospitals.

What does St. Francis Hospital gain from the consortium? A great deal of time is spent in meetings, such as administrators' and trustees' meetings once each month. The administrator feels that it is a waste of time, in part because he has heard the material several times, and he resents spending two mornings a month listening to material that he has heard before. Perhaps he expects too much from the consortium, but he does not feel he is getting his money's worth. He does not think that the consortium will grow in terms of strength or in terms of making an impact on anyone or anything. However, the other administrators seem to be satisfied with the way things are going, so it won't go away. He is not sure at some point whether or not St. Francis will withdraw, just on a monetary basis alone. He believes that one of the reasons it took a long time for all the hospitals to join the consortium was because they all knew that once they made the commitment, it would be very hard to withdraw, and it might give the hospital a bad name in the community. He no longer feels that it would make too much of an impact within the community if a hospital decided that it wanted to withdraw from the consortium. All in all, he feels that in this day and age hospitals have to work together as a group because if they do not pull together, they will get knocked down one by one. He does find it valuable to be able to talk to other administrators and other physicians. Physicians in the community should get to know one another in order to learn that they all have common problems, so in general a consortium is a good idea.

A physician from St. Francis Hospital, also on the professional staff council of the consortium, commented that the consortium has allowed open communication among the health care providers in the Hartford area. As a physician representative, it has been his responsibility to report to the St. Francis medical staff matters that are addressed at consortium meetings. He also attempts to expose the staff to the national scene that John Danielson is involved with. He believes that physicians, in general, are too enmeshed in their practices and are not interested or aware of what goes on in Washington. He admits that before joining the consortium, he was not aware of what hospital care involved in terms of costs and personnel and has gained a greater appreciation for the problems confronting hospital trustees and administrators. He believes that the greatest accomplishment of the consortium has been the opportunity to sit down and talk to one's colleagues.

A representative of the University of Connecticut School of Medicine noted that the consortium has expanded the number of hospital beds available for the extensive clinical programs at the undergraduate level of the medical school from 200 to 3000. One of the first problems the consortium dealt with was the number of graduates to be turned out every year and in what specialties. The consortium began to look at this issue, and its members agreed to limit the total number of graduates produced every year in psychiatry and surgery. In addition, the residency budgets of all the hospitals are now shared, and standardized salaries and fringe benefits for residents are being developed.

The greatest fear among the hospitals in the area is that the university will exclude them from the educational process, that is, graduate internship programs. In addition, the university has the power to withhold academic appointments. The greatest problem facing the consortium is that of proving itself to its members:

> The hospitals are entering a period of crisis. They must deal with cost control from state and federal governments. In this new era, will the Consortium be able to provide the hospitals with mechanisms to deal with cost controls? Will it make it possible for one hospital to cut down revenue and for another to raise it? Will it help them share facilities? These are the challenges facing the Consortium today.

A senior manager from Mt. Sinai Hospital and member of the management council of the consortium added a further factor to the three just mentioned as instrumental in the foregoing of the consortium: the presence of several new administrators without historical complicating relationships to tie them down.

One of the most important issues that the consortium addressed was the equality issue written into the bylaws:

> The equality statement in the bylaws is very important. It makes for a true partnership. Every hospital has three representatives. I think that is important. I think it is not only important from the point of view of each individual hospital, I think that equality among the trustees, doctors, and administrators is equally important. It does not make it a board dominated by either hospital administrators or by trustees, which is the case in some consortia. It makes it a true amalgamation of the traditional three elements in the management of a hospital.

One of the most difficult tasks in the initial stages of the consortium's development was having to "sell" it to the hospitals, particularly to the medical staffs. They had to persuade the staffs that it would give them an opportunity to plan and to act together; also, if the hospitals did not take the initiative in self-determination, the government would determine their future for them. Cooperation was inevitable in any event, and they were going to have to start working together.

The administrators produced a sharing document that showed all the interlocking relationships among the various institutions that already existed. There seemed to be enough need and concern that not one hospital was brave enough to stand up and say that they were against it, although there were a number of hospitals with medical staffs who were afraid of being swallowed up by the larger hospitals.

Group arrangements developed on a departmental basis, and senior staff from the social work departments, medical records, the communications, and ambulatory services started meeting on a regular basis. These activities kept everyone talking and so kept them from fighting.

> The deterrent effect of the Consortium is almost as valuable as its accomplishments. The fact that a department head would be embarrassed to think about doing something that exists elsewhere is as important as the fact that he sat down to talk to three of his colleagues at the other hospitals about doing something together.

The powers vested in the consortium are really powers of moral persuasion. There are no real powers as there are no sanctions. The consensus approach to decision making has been very important.

> I think the hospitals know that unless they get Consortium consensus and approval for particular programs, whether it be a programmatic idea or just a simple purchase of an elevator (which obviously has no planning implications for any other hospital), their own credibility is at stake, and hospitals are very jealous of their credibility. If they can't be believed, they are putting at risk much more important issues such as the quality of care and the management of the hospital and the fiduciary responsibility vested in the board. We are dealing with credibility. Every hospital comes and lays its credibility on the line before the Consortium, and if by consensus the Consortium would say "no," this would be an enormous deterrent.

This has not happened yet. What has occurred is that issues that are obviously going to be rejected by the board are first mentioned informally, and a message is usually sent to the hospital involved advising it to reconsider its request. Consequently, issues doomed to failure are rarely brought before the entire board.

The senior manager from Mt. Sinai views the role of John Danielson as a facilitator, planner, peacemaker, diplomat, politician, public relations person, and elder statesman. It is impossible to make all the people happy all the time, so he does pretty well. One of the problems is the lack of regularly obtainable, tangible results that one could demonstrate not only to oneself but to the outside world. He fears that the consortium will be so distracted by responding to government involvement that it won't really be able to do anything meaningful in terms of joint planning. Unless the consortium produces some results in filling the unmet needs in the community, then it will have failed in a very important responsibility. There is a whole group of people who are not getting the kind of care that they should, and the consortium should do something about it. While many are committed to the consortium, too many, especially doctors, are still parochially disinterested.

Over the next few years the consortium will remain an apolitical organization. It may make attempts to be a peacemaker, but in terms of accomplishments, he believes it will reach a plateau in terms of the number of things it can point to that it has accomplished. The number and type of activities the consortium will get into will depend primarily on external influences. There is not sufficient money in the system to stimulate a lot of growth within the hospitals to produce too many dynamic projects for the consortium to get involved with. However, if the reimbursement system changes over the period of the next four or five years, the consortium will have some significant activities to get involved with. What they do have is a mechanism in place that can react to the rapid changes in the evolution of health care. The investment that the community has made in the consortium has been and will continue to be worthwhile. To those who are interested in developing a consortium, he gives the following advice:

> The dynamics of the Hartford Consortium really are those which are necessary before you can put together a group of trustees or hospital administrators and say let's do joint planning. One either believes that diversity is healthy or one believes that we ned a uniform kind of system.
> I do not believe in a uniform kind of system; I do not believe that we need one health care model in the U.S., and if diversity is beneficial, then it has really been beneficial in this community. There is good medical care at a reasonable cost in this community. In addition, you need people meeting socially; you need the integration on the board levels; you need the hospital administrators feeling comfortable with each other and knowing each other by first name; you need the kind of basic trust that exists after some investment has been made. Now that does not mean that you cannot have a consortium without it. It means that you have got to create the appropriate environment if it does not exist. And you should not expect great wonders in a consortium that does not have it until you have created that atmosphere.

Chapter 9

Conclusions and Model

Chapters 9 and 10 present some conclusions to be derived from the case studies. Chapter 9 raises some specific issues: strategy, attitude change, managing collaboration, what can be expected from it, and how paradigmatic issues can be confronted and avoided. Then a five-stage model of process is presented. Leadership questions are discussed in chapter 10.

First the Newbury story is concluded, as it provides an opportunity to explore many of the concerns that bedevil those who try to create a climate for collaboration.

One thing must be emphasized: collaboration is rarely, if ever, voluntary. In spite of an increasingly complex, hostile, and rapidly changing environment for health institutions, which, some theorists say, requires collaboration for survival, rare is the statesman who undertakes a collaborative endeavor without needing to. Competitive and independent values die hard in this society. Therefore, collaboration will not come about through inertia or goodwill. It has to be managed.

Two threads run through the Newbury story. The problems of Community wax and wane, and the conditions for solution shift. The problems initially were clearly those of Community Medical Center alone, since Newbury Memorial felt that it was not part of the problem but only a possible and reluctant part of the solution. But the problem for Community Medical Center never seemed to force drastic remedies. The initial problem essentially was: could Community Medical Center, then St. Mary's, continue as a financially viable health institution primarily devoted to acute care in a community overbedded for acute care? The rational answer, repeatedly stated, was no. But this definition was emotionally rejected. It was not until late in the story that Memorial began to regard itself as part of the problem and not just part of the solution. The conditions for solution depend to some degree on the criticality of a problem, but largely lie in the attitudes of those parties who have to work together in any possible solution, namely, the trustees, the administrators, and the doctors.

Even when hospitals seek to collaborate, there appear to be inordinate difficulties. One set of problems derives from the traditional resource-rich, resource-poor relationship. Smaller hospitals approached by larger ones respond with suspicion and distrust: "They want to take over our patients." In town after town the story is how small hospitals prefer to refer patients to a city many miles away rather than a closer one because they know that their patients will have to come back if they travel far and are concerned that they may get gobbled up if the distance is too small.

What are the other fears? There is a fear of loss of power. There is a fear of loss of identity that may get swallowed up in that larger whole. An identity is not just a name, although that is important. When Affiliated Hospitals in Boston was thinking about getting three hospitals together, name was so important that they planned a building with three entrances, over which the three individual institutions would have their original names. There is also a fear among individuals, especially administrators, that they may lose career opportunities. There are many fears.

These fears are often exacerbated by a history of past overtures that have not led to anything and have become a tradition of bad faith. Often one institution has approached another about something and has been turned down. Perhaps repeatedly. Feelings build, and there comes a point when, although rationality may dictate the necessity to work together, distrust is of such a level that it is not conceivable.

HOW TO CREATE A CLIMATE FOR COLLABORATION

What does it take to bring together what may be long-time competitors or even enemies? Clearly it is harder to get collaboration if there is a past history of independence or even competitiveness, as is so often the case. It is easier if at least some of the institutions have either had complementary roles in the community or have even been linked together in some fashion.

If at least there are mechanisms that allow the parties to talk, and not just talk when there is a crisis or a problem to be faced, then there is the possibility of getting to know one another and diminishing historical distrust. Take parents and their adolescent children. They go their own ways: the parents are middle-aged, preoccupied with their careers and their social activities; the adolescents are preoccupied with their peers. Perhaps the only time they talk is when a problem comes up. It is hardly surprising that if this is the only occasion for significant conversation, the relationship deteriorates. Even in industry where managers are trained and supposedly sophisticated, appreciation of the need for mechanisms to keep conversation continuing is sparse. In a major consumer company, a manager of a service group met with his key colleagues only when there was a problem to be solved. It was hardly surprising that their relationship was colored by the fact that they always met only when there were difficulties to be diminished. It took a simple suggestion to state that perhaps they ought to talk regularly so that when problems came up, they could be handled in the context of a positive relationship.

It is important to deal with issues that might be of common interest and not wait for a crisis that forces a win-lose result. If possible problems are identified in advance and in a nonthreatening way and broader context, they can better be dealt with. They should be raised in a neutral fashion so that it does not become a matter of who is responsible for the problem or who is to blame for the lack of a solution.

Probably the most crucial thing that has to be faced as a collaborative relationship is considered is that the collaborative process has to be managed. It has been stated previously that no new paradigm will be entertained until the old is disproved and that paradigm shift is multidimensional and involves atitude and value change as a fundamental prerequisite.

MANAGING THE PROBLEMS: DISPROVING THE OLD PARADIGM

There are always problems that institutions have to face together when they consider collaboration, and these may continue at a level that is less than that forcing a serious approach to solution for a considerable time. Sometimes it may be necessary to precipitate a crisis so that one of the institutions becomes sufficiently concerned to enter in all seriousness into dialogue previously only toyed with. It was only when three successive consulting firms produced adverse reports followed by a deliberate intervention on the part of the State Health Department in the form of a new reimbursement system that was designed to drive out small hospitals, that Community Medical Center seriously considered some of the alternatives that were offered it. There are many ways to influence the severity of problems affecting health institutions such as through legislators or the reimbursement system or the health services agency that is responsible for planning. This is so important that it is almost a dictum that all the actors must hurt. If one of the actors doesn't hurt, if they feel they can go it alone, then collaboration becomes just about impossible because they do not need to engage in the often painful paradigm shift. Often one hospital may feel that it is in a position to go it alone, or that it could afford to let another go bankrupt and pick it up for less, or that it isn't their business, or that it is easier to do any of these than to get together and face some difficult joint decisions. Whether the actors hurt and how much is something that can be managed.

MANAGING CONDITIONS
FOR SOLUTION

A problem can continue indefinitely without the conditions for the possibility of solution being changed at all, i.e., without a new paradigm being readily apparent or accessible. Since an important aspect of resistance to paradigm shift is entrenched attitudes, often the conditions for solution lie in the attitudes of those with power, i.e., the attitudes of key trustees, administrators, and doctors. If there are significant people whose presence on the scene make it impossible for a form of collaboration to be realized, managing the conditions for solution means getting rid of them. In Newbury it was not until Gary Millen changed his board, removing those with historically built-up prejudices and parochial points of view, that the conditions for solution, namely, the readiness to take responsibility for the community and to make a reasonable offer to the small hospital, radically changed.

In general, two major figures seem to contribute toward creating a favorable climate and opportunity for successful collaboration. A highly regarded visionary helps. In Hartford, Connecticut, a senior physician with charisma and status in the community, two years from retirement, had a vision of how Hartford's health system might be and was instrumental in setting in motion the movement toward the Capital Area Health Consortium. The existence of a competent and experienced executive to run the collaborative enterprise who understands the processes that must be dealt with and who does not threaten the institution may be significant also. One can spot those hospital groups who intend to work together (and at what) and those who do not by the caliber and skill of their chosen group executive. In Hartford, the Capital Area Health Consortium chose an experienced hospital administrator. In Cambridge, Massachusetts, the South Middlesex Hospital Association chose a young planner, and the Cancer Collaboration Association chose a research physician.

Paradigm shift occurs only when an old paradigm will not work or a new one is better. Collaboration occurs only when competition fails or cooperation offers some overriding edge. Thus the major reasons for collaboration today tend to be the negative ones of cost pressure and threat from planning and regulatory activity and only occasionally the promise of a new vision. Most of the case studies fall into the first category. Hartford is an exception in the second. The significance of the able executive is that he sees what the new paradigm requires to be done, without symbolizing it, and thus he acts as a lightning rod for the emotions aroused by the loss of the original paradigm.

Paradigm renunciation is followed by setting the stage for a new paradigm, and the issue of value change has been raised. What values in particular?

The first value change is from short-term self-interest to a long-term enlightened value. Traditionally, many who run health institutions feel that their responsibility lies in the short-term well-being of their institution, a not unnatural and human concern. This view has led, in many instances, to contributing to urban blight by failure to accept any responsibility for the physical or social conditions of a neighborhood lying outside the immediate walls of such an institution. The results are all too obvious in all too many cities—staff who risk mugging on their way to work and the flight to the suburbs. On the other hand, an enlightened administrator in Green Bay, Wisconsin, decided to spend discretionary dollars on improving the parking lot in the pleasant middle-class urban neighborhood surrounding his hospital, as a foresighted avoidance of a similar future fate.

A second attitude shift is from parochialism to societal responsibility. The former attitude expresses, "I do not have to be bothered since it isn't my business." The Newbury Memorial trustees by and large felt that their responsibility was to the mission of Newbury Memorial, namely, protecting its excellent reputation as an acute-care institution. Taking on anything else would dilute this mission. The change in this attitude, which had its beginning in the later meeting of the joint committee and was highlighted by Heller's January 1978 letter to the trustees and the community, was enhanced with the installation of a new, younger board of trustees and was further enhanced by the actions of the HSA in requiring that planning involve all those in a community and not just sections of it. People came to realize that the Community Medical Center was a problem for the entire community and not just for Community Medical Center itself. Another aspect of this attitude shift is from position taking to problem solving.

Finally, there is the need to separate rationality from emotion if problems are to be solved. As long as feelings run high as data are exchanged, data merely becomes ammunition in a protracted debilitating war. Despite a flow of financial figures for over a decade, the problem of Community Medical Center's situation could never produce any resolution until the emotional investment of the public and the medical community on the subject was separated out. Problems are so often treated as rational when in fact they are highly charged emotionally. Only when feelings have been acknowledged and dealt with can the rational aspect be realized! Thus it is probably helpful for the stronger party in a collaborative venture to be explicit about their knowledge and understanding of the weaker party's real fears and to satisfy them both by demonstrating awareness and understanding and by taking appropriate action to relieve the fears. If both of these steps are not taken, then the chances are that collaboration will be difficult to get off the ground. For this reason it is probably important to start with relatively trivial issues to demonstrate and work through the early emotion-laden issues that will be identified later under the discussion of stages. Working through these issues over trivial concerns builds trust, which then can be tested when the more difficult decisions have to be faced later. For example, it might be tactical for the stronger members of the future collaboration to encourage the weaker to organize together before the total grouping is formed so that they will be in a position of strength to deal with the strong members. Indeed, this approach is used in some business situations in which management or corporations prefer to deal with strong unions rather than weak ones because of the divisiveness of the weak ones who cannot make decisions and stick to them.

NEWBURY REVISITED

Entrenched attitudes have underlain much of the Newbury story but have rarely or ever been made explicit in it. One anecdote has an assistant administrator from Newbury Memorial attending a St. Patrick's Day Irish Catholic cocktail party and, upon being introduced, receiving boos from those present. Some Jewish doctors refused by Memorial became intensely loyal to the Catholic hospital that opened its doors to them. Part of St. Mary's continued existence ironically lay in the never-spoken economics of the fact that many of the subspecialists at Newbury Memorial needed referrals from the primary-care physicians at Community Medical Center and could not afford to see them go.

Initially, the overtures from St. Mary's to Newbury Memorial were perfectly rationally rejected, but these rejections led to more entrenched attitudes that made further resolution even more difficult. Memorial's protective attitudes led to restraint and to imply rejection of St. Mary's physicians when only a few were in question. This uncorrected implication probably underlay much of the later doctor resistance.

As St. Mary's became Community Medical Center and tried to position itself to become more attractive to Newbury Memorial, paradoxically it incurred debts that worsened its problems, and at the same time Memorial's own growth reduced the need for Community Medical Center as an acute-care facility. The problem thus got worse. As Community Medical Center's problems worsened, Memorial became more and more concerned that the smaller hospital, if acquired, would become a financial albatross around its neck.

However, there were some slight shifts in the conditions for solution. A joint committee began talking to each other and thus built confidence, while the two administrators, Carl Metcalf and Gary Millen, developed a day-to-day working relationship on what they saw as a community problem. Fred Manzelli was slowly edging his board at Community Medical Center toward a realistic appreciation of Community's problems, and weaning them away from a slavish support of the medical staff's adamant opposition to anything but the continuation of St. Mary's in acute care. The new, smaller Memorial board recognized its responsibility to the larger community rather than to its own interests as in the past, and when fully informed of the problems, the potential for solution and actions needed, was able to act in a well-informed manner and with dispatch.

The problem for Community Medical Center deteriorated with

each of three successive consulting reports, but here was an argument as to the need to distinguish rationality from emotionalism. At least these three shocks did help Fred Manzelli to move his trustees toward some compromise solution. The doctors' resistance, eroded by the waning support of the trustees, was finally finished off by Bob Dickinson's revelations, freeing up the possibility of alternative solutions not before available.

Both the Department of Health and the HSA, as outside actors, played key roles in this evolving process. The Department of Health exacerbated the problems by creating a reimbursement system that made it impossible for Community Medical Center as an under-utilized facility and consequently a high-cost operation to exist as an acute-care institution. It also offered favorable financial terms to Memorial if they should be willing to pick up Community Medical Center's debt. Thus they made the problem worse and therefore more needy of attention, and improved the possibility of solution by significantly relieving Memorial of an important impediment.

Alan Hadley at the HSA also emphasized Community Medical Center's plight by reiterating that there was no place for it as an acute-care facility, while again facilitating and supporting the Health Department's creation of a possible solution.

The final factor, although small, was the entry of Crandall Hospital and the development of a consortium with Memorial that made the alternative uses proposed by the HSA economically viable when they might have been marginally interesting to Memorial alone.

CANCER COLLABORATION ASSOCIATION AND STRATEGY

The central purpose of program collaboration is the improvement of service. A review of the Cancer Collaboration Association (CCA) strategy in attempting this follows. Improvement involves improving linkages among institutions since single institutions cannot effectively meet all needs. Issues to be considered include:

Given that the medical system is made up of a large number of institutions including, for example, acute-care hospitals, long-term and convalescent institutions as well as community agencies, what parts of the system should join together?

Are the existing connections among the institutions adequate or should new connections be established?

Should an organization be set up that is separate from the hospitals themselves?

If a new and separate organization is established, should it play a consulting or facilitative role, a directive role, a coordinating role, or some combination of these?

If a new and separate organization is established, what kind of structure should it have so that it can best achieve its objectives?

It is obvious in reviewing the history of the CCA, particularly the hiring of staff, the kinds of activities that the staff has been involved in, that the key decisions concerned choosing between a large number of available options. A certain strategy is implicit in these decisions whether it was made explicit or not. Some of the rejected alternatives were the following:

Preliminary collaboration could have occurred between the Cancer Control Center and the initiating hospital.

Extended care and municipal institutions could have been included as well as acute-care hospitals.

The Cancer Control Center could have refused to take a leading role in the early collaborative efforts.

Rather than hiring staff at all, representatives from each member institution might have donated their time.

While it is quite possible to work directly with hospitals, the goal of upgrading care may be facilitated by the development of a separate organization whether for specific disease category such as cancer or for more general reasons such as planning and administrative purposes (e.g., a hospital consortium). Any group concerned with the goal of upgrading care has to develop an explicit strategy for achieving it. Any strategy essentially takes the form of making a choice among the following options:

1. To work directly with the health system.
2. To work with an existing multi-institutional organization where it exists.
3. To set up a new multi-institutional organization.

In this example it would have been possible to have worked with the first hospital when approached by them and/or with other institutions on an individual basis to encourage the development of linkages. Extension could have taken the form either of informal linkages or contractual arrangements. One might have taken an existing multi-institutional organization, such as a small grouping of physicians who had been meeting for some time prior to the formation of the CCA and had worked with it as a coordinating body. What was in fact decided was to set up a new multi-institutional organization called the Cancer Collaboration Association.

Having made the decision to work with some kind of multi-institutional organization, further issues have to be faced:

Should a multi-institutional organization have its own staff or not?
Should the staff be drawn from member institutions or from other sources?
Should the resources in addition to staff—namely, money and space—be part of member institutions or separate from them?

The pros and cons obviously include some key issues, such as:

Would the nascent multi-institutional organization become captured by some particular element of the health system, or
Could it be helped to remain natural?

Given these initial decisions, further critical ones may briefly be mentioned. What is the purpose in setting up a multi-institutional organization? Is it to stimulate the service system to develop linkages, is it to stimulate new activities, or is it to set up the multi-institutional organization as an end in itself, as a political forum in which attitudes might be altered? These are all reasonable but different purposes and need articulated since the activities that are necessary to implement them are clearly different.

The roles and relationships of staff to the multi-institutional organization—in this case, the CCA—have to be clearly articulated, established, and implemented. There are various alternatives:

The staff of the multi-institutional organization may be permanent or temporary. This choice may be made at the beginning, or it may change over time.
The role of the external organization—in this case, the CCA—staff may take a variety of forms. Should the staff undertake activities or work with other community groups? For example, should their role be to educate the public, or should that job fall entirely to some other body? Should they develop standards of care or should the PSRO do this, in as much as they are already developing such standards? Should the CCA be a corporate head to its member institutions, which might be considered "divisions," or should it serve as a consultant or a catalyst?

Finally, it is only proper to point out that the CCA is being put under the microscope at a point only two years at most from inception. Collaboration is still at a very early stage. And while these issues can be raised, these same issues were still largely unresolved in the South Middlesex Hospital Association at a later time—some three years after inception—and are even lurking in the Capital Area Health Consortium, supposedly at a still later stage of collaboration, after some four years. Clearly, competition and independence die hard, and the collaboration paradigm is difficult to bring about, at least through the intermediate type of structure such as a consortium.

SOUTH MIDDLESEX
HOSPITAL ASSOCIATION

Like many other consortia, the South Middlesex Hospital Association is an example of the early stages of the development of collaborative relationships. It had no prototype to model itself after and has consequently evolved through trial-and-error learning. Its actual achievements have been few. The common opinion of many of the participants has been,

> At least individuals from various institutions have gotten to know each other, and an institutional forum for meeting each other and for sharing information exists.

It appears that while there have been many barriers to the development of the collaborative processes at the SMHA, there have been few facilitators. In fact, it seems that the multiplicity of barriers has itself been responsible for the paucity of facilitators.

Some of the barriers to the development of the collaborative processes in the external environment include (1) the lack of clarity regarding the time when the HSA would become powerful, and (2) the lack of direct incentives to foster multi-institutional collaboration.

Some of the barriers from within the association include the following: (1) the long history of competition among the member hospitals; (2) the overbedding and duplication of certain services within the SMHA area; (3) a certain imbalance in the competitive strengths of the rival hospitals, e.g., Cambridge City and Mt. Auburn; (4) conflicting interests between the hospitals' needs and the needs of the community; (5) the lack of physician involvement in the association's activities; (6) the lack of leadership; and (7) the diversity among the types of hospitals involved in the association that may account for the lack of mutual interests and concerns.

The facilitators to the development of the collaborative processes in the external environment have been: (1) the legislative mandate for the development of multi-institutional arrangements, and (2) the increasing federal and state regulations that have tightened resources for the expansion of health facilities.

Some of the facilitators within the association include: (1) the desire on the part of the members to become acquainted with one another and to share information to a limited degree, and (2) the establishment of the key committees.

In addition, several other factors must be taken into consideration. First, the SMHA has not had an experienced executive director. Second, the association has not been able to facilitate the awarding of multi-institutional medical staff privileges. Third, the majority of the discussions at the board meetings have centered around building external ties and countering external threats, rather than resolving internal conflicts. Fourth, in terms of dealing with internal issues, the members have focused primarily on nonthreatening substantive matters—e.g., the coordination of bioengineering repairs, credit collection, and personnel services—instead of dealing with the more important matters—e.g., the purpose of the consortium, the decision-making mechanism, and sources of multi-institutional conflicts. If the barriers are many and the facilitators few, making a success of the consortium will take a long time. A speedier progress must involve a conscious effort to reduce the barriers and to increase the facilitators. Consequently, a greater stress should be placed on discussing process issues and resolving the internal conflicts.

The association currently uses a voting procedure to arrive at consortium decisions. This procedure is followed at all levels—in board meetings, in committee meetings, and in the task forces. A voting procedure prevents the development of internal commitment by member institutions to consortium decisions. It might be preferable to supplement the formal voting procedure with a conscious attempt to arrive at significant decisions on a consensual basis. A consensus mechanism may also facilitate the discussion of threatening issues because individuals would feel secure in the knowledge that no decision would be forced on them. For such a mechanism to work, however, it is essential that the executive director be a competent facilitator. Some of the key tasks that he should perform are to (1) facilitate a discussion of process issues; (2) help resolve multi-institutional conflicts; and (3) enable the carrying out of programmatic planning.

In addition, the executive director must make a conscious attempt to help the institutional representatives realize that they bear the primary responsibility for making the consortium a success or failure. If at any time the consortium seems to be failing, the executive director should refrain from shifting the primary responsibility to himself because this would lead to a further decline in the internal commitment by member institutions toward the consortium. All critical consortium decisions should be implemented not by the executive director but by the hospital representatives toward consortium decisions. Consensual decision making, discussion of process issues, and conversion of private knowledge into public knowledge are a few of the key ingredients necessary for generating this type of commitment.

CAPITAL AREA HEALTH CONSORTIUM

The Capital Area Health Consortium is in some ways a pivotal case. As an early and apparently successful prototype, it has been regarded as a model by many. But the issue regarding the concrete achievements of the consortium seems to elicit mixed responses not only from the different individuals but very often from the same individuals. On the one hand, the members of the consortium seem to have positive feelings toward the collaborative activities the consortium decided to undertake. However, they also stated that in terms of concrete achievements, there was really not much to show and that achievements have primarily been in "bringing trustees, administrators, and physicians from the various institutions together, and thus providing a forum for them to share their problems and their ideas with each other."

The principal cause of this paradox appears to be the possibility that a good many of the collaborative activities would have been undertaken even without the consortium. This has led some trustees to wonder whether the consortium has served any purpose at all. One could hypothesize that the consortium caused such activities to be undertaken sooner and with much less stress. One may also question whether the autonomy and competence of each institution has been preserved to a greater extent than would be the case if the consortium had not existed. The following decisions and/or activities do appear to have been influenced or brought about by the consortium:

1. The establishment of a system of consortium-affiliated medical staff to regulate the award of interinstitutional staff privileges to physicians.
2. The coordination of medical education, that is, having consortium-wide residency programs.

3. The sharing of facilities and a radiologist in the field of radiation therapy.
4. An earlier postponement by St. Francis Hospital of its CAT-scanner application for one year. Also the current agreement between the various consortium institutions that all of them can make use of the body scanners at Hartford and St. Francis Hospitals and the brain scanner at New Britain General Hospital.
5. The endorsement by the consortium of Hartford Hospital's application for renovation of its obstetrics facilities.
6. The agreement between Hartford and St. Francis Hospitals that Hartford's open heart surgery team will make use of the facilities at St. Francis.
7. The consortium's decision to make a rehabilitation center of of Newington's Children's Hospital.
8. The consortium's decision to base neonatology at the University of Connecticut School of Medicine.

The preceding list would tend to suggest that the consortium does have some concrete achievements to show in terms of outcome measures. However, it also shows that really difficult issues such as closing down or converting excess obstetrics and pediatric beds have not yet been tackled. Some of the reasons may be: (1) the Capital Area does not suffer from major, clear-cut, undisputed overbedding and duplication of services, and the excess of facilities that actually exist are not perceived as crucial factors in any self-assessment of the consortium's progress. (2) Issues dealing with the closure of existing facilities are perceived as very threatening to certain individuals, and it is believed that the consortium needs some more time to develop enough maturity so that these threatening issues can be confronted. By contrast, issues that deal with the location of new facilities are not perceived as threatening as long as the norm of fairness is satisfied. (3) there does not seem to be any imminent HSA pressure to close down any existing facilities. Perhaps some of the reasons for the dissatisfaction among some of the individuals within the consortium is that the consortium did not deal with the concrete issue of excess facilities.

A barrier of importance included a keen sense of competitive self-interest, and there is no evidence that this has changed at all. There were facilitators that existed prior to the formation of the consortium, and their confluence led to the conception of the consortium toward the end of 1972. Progress of the consortium after the idea was conceived has depended on the extent to which the barriers have been broken down or kept in check and the facilitators developed. In regard to the development of facilitators, it would appear that the consortium has made significant progress:

1. A conscious decision was made to call the consortium a "Health Consortium" rather than a "Hospital Consortium.' This seems to symbolize a desire to develop a consumer orientation rather than an institutional orientation for the consortium.
2. There was a conscious decision to actively involve all three constituencies such as the trustees, the administrators, and the physicians in the system.
3. A highly experienced and competent "process facilitator" in the form of John Danielson was hired to be the consortium's executive director.
4. A set of consortium-affiliated medical staff bylaws were adopted to facilitate the awarding of interinstitutional medical staff privileges.
5. A decision was made to adopt a "programmatic" rather than an ad hoc approach for the generation and discussion of issues.
6. A decision was made to arrive at all significant substantive decisions on a consensual basis.

The decision to operate through four councils (the management, professional staff, hospital trustee, and council on education and research) appears to have been a useful method for focusing efforts. In addition, the establishment of numerous standing committees and ad hoc committees appears to have been a useful structure in order to deal with several issues at the same time and involve all the relevant people in the discussion on particular issues. Given the large number of the standing and ad hoc committees, it appears that the executive director could not serve as the driving force behind all of them. Consequently, it was necessary for the committee participants to begin to develop internal committees to making these committees a success.

The use of a programmatic approach for the generation and discussion of substantive issues has the advantage of bringing out gaps in the existing subsystem such as the rehabilitation of cardiac patients. This makes it easy for specific institutions, as well as the consortium, to provide rational arguments in support of Certificate of Need applications. By dealing with consumer benefit values, it makes it more likely that member institutions may agree to close down and/or relocate some of their existing services, and it provides a rational framework for involving health providers serving the same geographic area. The programmatic approach is a good facilitator, but its success would depend on the weaknesses and strengths of the other barriers and facilitators within the system.

The use of a consensus mechanism for making significant decisions has a number of advantages:

1. It helps keep the medical school and the VA Hospital within the consortium.
2. It allows threatening issues to be discussed.
3. It helps develop an internal commitment by the member institutions to consortial decisions.

The key tasks that the executive director needs to perform seem to be:

1. To facilitate a discussion of process issues and the carrying out of self-assessments.
2. Helping resolve interinstitutional conflicts and facilitate consensual decision making.
3. To enable the carrying out of programmatic planning.

It appears that John Danielson was fully aware of these requirements and was perceived by almost all the consortium members as being competent in meeting these requirements.

It does not seem, however, that the executive director alone can provide a sum total of leadership for the consortium. Until recently, the founder and a few other individuals played a very important role in the leadership function. Many of these individuals have left or are in the process of leaving. It is not unlikely that the new people may not have the same kind of identification with the consortium or a similar vision about its future. In this respect, the current situation is a test of the consortium's maturity. If the consortium is able to socialize the new people into its process effectively, then it might be able to use them as committed facilitators to its development. Otherwise, the risks of their remaining either neutral or as barriers to the consortium's development are high. If such a creation of new facilitators can help the consortium ride over the loss of leaders like the first president and others, it would demonstrate that it has a life of its own and and is not dependent on the presence of certain key individuals. That is the criterion for institutional maturity.

However, an epilogue must, in all honesty, be appended, and it is this which forces skepticism about all forms of collaboration short of merger. John Danielson has left, and in his wake one of the larger hospitals, originally most committed, is considering going its competitive way as there is little or nothing to keep it within the consortium. Thus an existing enterprise has existed as long as the idea that fueled it, but because nothing fundamental had changed, its stability was always, no matter what publicly showed, fragile.

A MODEL OF DEVELOPMENTAL STAGES OF COLLABORATION

In this model, derived from the case studies and from other work over the years, five stages of the development of collaboration are suggested, and issues are described for each stage. These issues represent tasks that must be faced and dealt with if the collaboration is to proceed successfully.

Stage 1: Forming the Multi-institutional System

The earliest questions that the initiators of the idea to set up a multi-institutional system need to resolve are:

Which specific organizations should be invited to join?
What should the statement of purpose be?

In fact, these questions are interactive and need to be answered simultaneously.

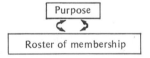

Given a particular formulation of purpose, one can logically deduce the list of organizations that should be a part of the collaboration. By contrast, it is conceivable that independent factors may bring about a particular set of institutions. In such an event, the purpose would evolve from what the institutional representatives seem to agree on.

Situation-specific characteristics thus seem to play a major role in how the purpose and the roster of membership evolve. What does not seem to be situation specific, however, is a normative statement of the long-term direction in which this evolution should proceed.

As this research indicates, hospitals get together because they hope that they can retain a greater control over their autonomy in the face of increasing governmental regulations and be more effective in dealing with these regulators. One effective way in which a group of hospitals can gain collective control over their collective destiny in the face of increasing governmental regulation is by being instrumental in the forging of a health care system rather than a nonsystem of fragmented services.

Thus one valid statement of long-term purpose appears to be: "We aim to forge a health care system in this area." If such is a statement of effective long-term purpose, then in the long run, all institutions that would be critical to such a health care system must be part of the collaboration.

A long-term vision of purpose and membership, however, can at best be only a guide to more short-term decisions. Situation-specific factors will have a significant bearing on these decisions. The most relevant criterion for short-term decisions on purpose and membership seem to be: "Strengthen the facilitators and weaken the barriers to the development of collaborative relationships—at least until the collaboration builds up a critical momentum of its own." One major step toward meeting this criterion is the development of norms among the institutional representatives whereby these individuals regard each other and their institutions as strong, competent, and equal. Viewed from this perspective, the leadership should avoid creating a situation in which one particular institution is viewed as a burden on other institutions. In other words, institutions that are weak—either because of competence of finances—should not be invited in; or if they are, then the stronger institutions must be willing to assist the weaker institutions to become strong. This logic should be of specific relevance when the leaders of strong, big institutions are in the process of deciding whether some of the weak, small institutions should be invited in or not. In such situations, the decision often rests with the representatives of the strong, big hospitals. On their part, smaller regional hospitals are expected to be wanting to join the consortium anyway out of fear that by not joining they might eventually suffer; moreover, once they have joined, they may feel that their competence is not respected.

Looking at the evolution of the three consortium cases described, all include acute-care hospitals, whether small and weak, or large and successful hospitals. One of them appears to have developed more effectively than the others. One of the important reasons for this difference seems to be the fact that in the more successful consortium, CAHC, norms of strength, competence, equality, and respect have been built up and developed through concrete events; by contrast, in the less successful consortia, these norms have not been given much significance, indeed, were undermined in one case when it was at first proposed that the smaller regional hospitals be given one vote to the larger hospitals' three each. In the CCA it is not at all clear that the development of a sense of purpose by the nine hospitals has yet been achieved. This may be because beyond the rhetorical statements about upgrading cancer care, the real issues have not been confronted, especially where confrontation means policing poor quality care. It has been assumed that the CCA would never play a policing role. Consequently, quality of care became part of the educational effort, and the possibility of effective action (that is, stage 3) was significantly reduced, since those physicians not adhering to adequate treatment standards would ignore the new standards, and those physicians who did adhere to adequate standards would in any case abide by them. The importance of a sense of purpose is that it is something with which they can all identify and thus transcend their differences in terms of needs and disparate facilities, while at the same time taking these differences into account. While the improvement of cancer treatment in the CCA and the facilitation of patient entry and treatment at all disease stages was of interest to the institutions, at least in a purely verbal form, it seems clear that:

These wishes were present before CCA came into existence.

No strategy was devised or implemented to address these wishes.

No leader emerged who was willing to operationalize words such as "quality of care" or "patient needs" in a way that could be acted on by the participants.

Stage 2: Developing the Infrastructure

Once a multi-institutional system has been formed, either formally or informally, the basic issue is: Which individuals will relate to each other and how? More specifically:

Which individuals from the member institutions should be invited to participate in the collaborative decision-making process?

What forums/committees should be created where these individuals can meet on an ongoing basis?

In the event of conflicts of loyalty/opinion on the part of two or more of the institutional representatives, how should these conflicts be resolved or not resolved and decisions made?

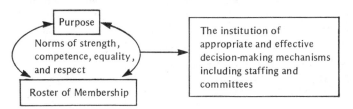

This phase is crucial, especially in mergers, since the potential loss of old identity with no new one yet emerging means a heightened need for some anchors as well as expression of mourning. Anchors may well take the form of a transitional structure and/or process that is to be trusted as the new shape forms. No trust, no progress. Staffing design is critical in consortia.

The CCA institutions failed to tackle some questions of concern. Should the CCA staff feel a responsibility to confront member institutions about their responsibility to think through the issues of upgrading care or about the consequences of policing versus not policing conformity to standards? i.e., should they lead or follow? If the CCA believes itself to be a defensive counterplanning hospital body with educational goals, should the CCA staff accept this, challenge it, or seek support within the community to give the hospitals increased leverage? In short, do CCA staff "belong" to the hospitals, are they an independent group, or are they partly responsive to the interests of the community and partly directed by the CCA? These issues will obviously influence their predilections for certain kinds of activities. Further issues to be faced regarding staff include: How many, where do they sit, who pays them, what skills and experience should they have, whom should they report to, and what should they do. All these have consequences and implications. Most of these are obvious; yet in many (most?) collaborative endeavors, little careful thought is given to staffing.

From the literature on organization theory, one can deduce the following theoretical guideline for the creation of appropriate and effective decision-making mechanisms:

> The differentiation in the structure used for multi-institutional decision making should match the diversity in the levels across which individual institutions need to interact and in the issues that are expected to be up for joint decision making.

It hardly needs mentioning that the three elements of any hospital are: trustees, administrators, and physicians. All three groups have considerable strategic power within each organization. It is therefore necessary that individuals from these three constituencies in every hospital interact with their counterparts from the other hospitals. Within this context, the theoretical guideline stated previously suggests the nature of appropriate decision-making mechanisms.

Accordingly, in many successful health collaborations, such as a consortium, the board consists of a trustee, the administrator, and the chief of medical staff from each institution. Furthermore, three standing committees of board members of the consortium exist—one of trustees, one of administrators, and one of the medical chiefs. The administrative and the medical committees may further set up task forces to examine key issues individually.

It seems clear that, whatever decision-making ability the CCA board had when it consisted of four institutions, it lost a good deal when it grew so radically from four to nine. Since no effective executive decision-making subgroup was formed, the result was lack of direction and reduced participation. The formation of a truly effective executive committee must of course be based on a trusting relationship on the part of all member institutions so that their best interests will at least be kept in mind, whether or not their representative sits on the executive committee. A decision-making mechanism that will ensure the development of purpose is crucial, e.g., voting as a mechanism can imply that a negative vote allows a hospital to opt out. Consensus, however, requires commitment. The key issues of purpose and action require the development of consensus in order to obtain commitment. Yet the policy board still votes. It is not clear what form the decision-making mechanism will take in the CCA, but it is clear that some decisions that appear to be consensual on the part of the policy board have not been implemented in the member institutions and that commitment at some basic level is absent.

Finally, competitive roles must be dealt with. These form the basis for the observation that people who represent institutions in an interinstitutional organization play dual roles or have multiple constituencies as responsible members of their own institution and as executives in an interinstitutional organization. At times, decisions may be required that place them in a potentially conflicting situation. Unless they have dealt with these dual roles, have thought about the consequences of this problem in terms of action, and unless they have established relationships of trust and power with their own constituencies at home, it is at this point that the interinstitutional organization will begin to crumble. As one might expect, it is clear that some administrators will not take on medical staffs.

Stage 3: Taking Concrete Action

A multi-institutional system exists to get things done. Accordingly, the basic issues at this stage are:

> What mix of activities should the collaboration take up for concrete collaborative action?

In what order should these activities be taken up?

Are activities nonparadigmatic, i.e., new or non-threatening, or paradigmatic, i.e., raising questions about a total realignment of the member institutions?

From all the possible activities, the leadership must help participants select a subset in which priorities reflect the overall purposes of the multi-institutional system. These activities must be backed up by commitment from the participants. The member institutions must act according to these priorities and be willing to sanction those members who do not. This commitment may take the form of backing up difficult actions, of committing resources, or of committing time. It may also include securing stability for the collaboration by obtaining long-term funding—another form of commitment. The appropriateness of the mechanisms of decision making developed in stage 2 will be reflected in the quality of the action taken in stage 3.

The process of sorting out priorities for action may well begin with a decision to use a "programmatic approach" for the generation and discussion of substantive issues. Under this approach, a particular program such as rehabilitation/cardiac care/cancer care is take up for scrutiny in its entirety. This helps focus attention on the rehabilitation of all aspects of health-care delivery within that particular program. Benefits are many:

It helps bring out gaps in the existing system.

It helps specific institutions and the multi-institutional organization in providing rational arguments in support of CON applications to fill these gaps.

By appealing to consumer-benefit values, it makes it a trifle more likely that member institutions may agree to close down/relocate some of their existing services.

It provides a rational framework for involving health providers serving the same geographic area but officially not within the multi-institutional organization.

If a decision to use the "programmatic approach" has been made, the next step would be to decide on which programs to take up for concrete decisions/action. This decision should be based on a judgment of the historical barriers and facilitators to the development of collaborative processes existing within the consortium and its environment. The "program" chosen should provide valuable experience to the consortium in using the "programmatic approach"; on the other hand, it should not be too explosive, otherwise the consortium may fall apart before any concrete learning has taken place. The revised sequence of activities now looks like Figure 9.1.

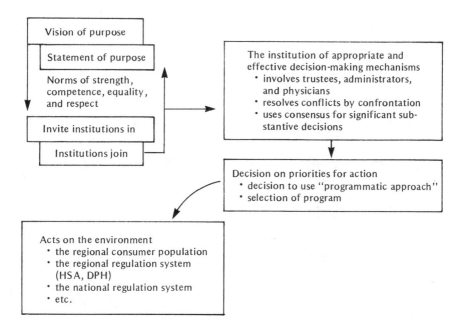

Espousing the need for a successful health collaboration and creating one through concrete action are two very different phenomena. In the short run, some institutional leaders may have to "bite the bullet," i.e., forgo short-run benefits for their institutions in return for greater long-term autonomy from regulatory agencies. The tendency may be to avoid doing so by picking up trivial "programs" for concrete action during the initial phases or new activities that do not raise questions of realignment. While this makes a collaborative setting less threatening to member institutions, it also breeds frustration and makes it increasingly difficult to tackle the more conflict-ridden "programs." After having begun with relatively trivial "programs," most collaborations have been found to undergo a period of crisis in which the participants feel very frustrated with the achievements of the organization. Progress will occur only if the "hurt" of not going ahead (threat of bankruptcy, loss of service, etc.) is less than the discomfort of proceeding. All members must "hurt" for matters to proceed, i.e., the old paradigm must be discounted for the new to be adopted. In many collaborations there is failure to progress at this point because:

No sanctions evolve for actions on the part of individual institutions
that would encourage cooperation with the goals of the group.

The low level of commitment on the part of memberships leads to
little or no confronting behavior; thus issues remain superficial
and noncontroversial.

Each institution is anxious to maintain the status quo and acts to
ensure that its own interests will not be subsumed by the
interests of the whole, a totally essential paradigmatic shift.

Examples are the SMHA and the CCA. The CAHC, when regarded
critically, is one also.

Stage 4: Vertical Integration

Stage 4 involves moving beyond collaboration to some structural and
process alteration that involves reallocating resources more efficiently toward redefined goals. This is a commitment to a new
paradigm and will generally only be true of those types of collaboration of the closer kind, i.e., merger types. This stage is somewhat
hypothetical, as relatively few mergers have proceeded this far,
although United Hospitals in St. Paul, Minnesota, is an example (see
Figure 9.1). Where there is reallocation of resources, there must be
some form of vertical integration, and in the environmental conditions earlier described, this is most likely to take the form of the
creation of an interorganizational matrix. There will of course be
some centralization of some functions. Probably also there is likely
to be a redefinition of the market in the light of the enhanced
capability of the aggregated and redeployed resources. Thus, for
example, Baptist Hospital in Memphis, Tennessee, when it joined a
group of equally large hospitals, now considers its catchment area to
be as far south as New Orleans, 400 miles away, a considerable
enlargement over the previously thought of market.

Why will vertical integration probably take the form of a matrix?
The matrix is the preferred structural choice when three basic
conditions exist simultaneously.[1] These conditions are:

1. *Pressures for shared resources.* Where organizations are under
considerable pressure to achieve economies of scale and high
performance utilizing scarce human resources and meeting high
quality standards, there is a clear indication to adopt a matrix.
2. *Pressures for high information-processing capacity.* If the demands placed on the organization are changing and relatively
unpredictable and therefore large amounts of new information
must be assimilated and responded to in a coherent way, such

uncertainty in the external environment calls for an enriched information-processing capacity within the organization. The more interdependence there is among people, as in criterion 1, the greater the information-processing load. Uncertainty, complexity, and interdependence all generate a need for information-processing capacity, which is enhanced by the matrix form of organization. This is not simply a matter of increasing the flow of reports, briefings, and informal communications through the information system, but weighing the significance of the new information and making decisions that commit the organization to a successfully adaptive response. More people must be in a position to think and act as general managers, and this is the kind of behavior that can result only from the matrix form of structure.

3. *Pressures for dual focus.* Finally, where organizations have outside pressures for dual focus, the matrix is the preferred form. In health as in aerospace, there is a need to focus both on the customer or patient and on complex, technical issues.

All these pressures have been discussed earlier. They all clearly indicate a need for a matrix form as the preferred structural form.

Stage 5: Growing

The basic issues here are:

When should new activities be taken up? How should they be selected?

Should new members be invited in? How should they be selected?

Here the "programmatic approach" comes in very handy, as it provides a rational framework not only to decide on what new activities but also to decide on what new members. The only critical decisions that the consortium members have to take deal with are, "when do we add on a new program?" After that, the process of using the programmatic approach may itself help the consortium in making decisions on new activities/new members.

The key consideration in addressing the issue of sequence is how each decision affects the ultimate purpose of the multi-institutional organization. This sense of purpose will determine who belongs. As the purpose changes over time, considerations of membership will also change. Participants should be aware that sequencing is difficult because of what has already happened between those who have joined colors, what might happen to those who are in the process, or who are considering it.

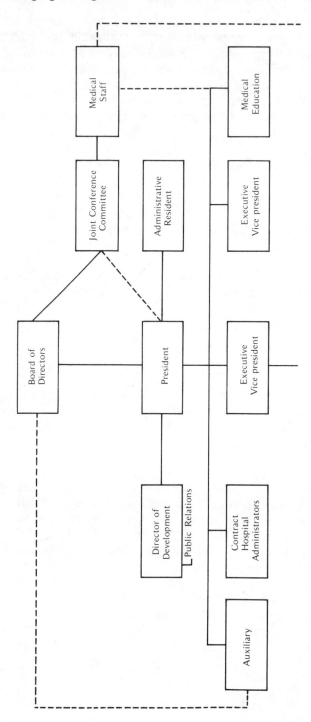

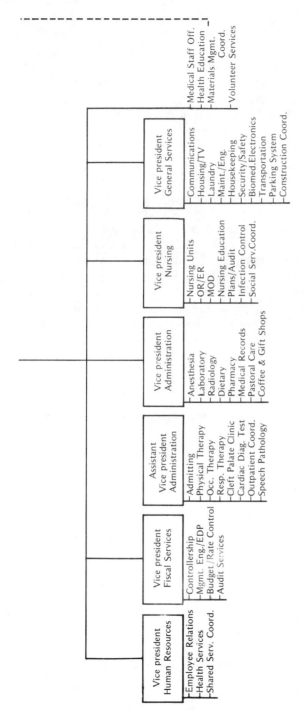

Figure 9.1. United Hospitals, Inc., St. Paul, Minnesota: Organization chart.

Initially, the four acute-care central hospitals chose to enlarge the CCA to nine by adding the five rural acute-care hospitals rather than move from acute-care activities to aftercare activities. This would have implied the need to add non-acute institutions, which would have been a reason for not choosing this route. It is interesting to note that there seemed to be little interest in bringing in other institutions in the area and no concern had been expressed about how they would be brought in, especially given the ostensible purposes of the collaboration. Again in the SMHA there was foot dragging about involving the non-acute facilities. Clearly, the ultimate goal is to improve the quality and quantity of links between resources and market. But should the early links be between those resource-rich institutions (the providers) to achieve rationalization and collaboration? Or should they be created among resource-poor institutions (the consumers)? Should they be formed directly with the market, that is, the patients themselves, to obtain better definitions of need? In the CCA the strategy was to induce cooperation among the resource-rich institutions.

To sum up, the evolutionary sequence of a successful health collaboration is expected to proceed as shown on the facing page with one caution: Often stage 4 is skipped or never reached.

NOTE

1. S.M. Davis and P.R. Lawrence, *Matrix* (Reading, Mass.: Addison-Wesley, 1977).

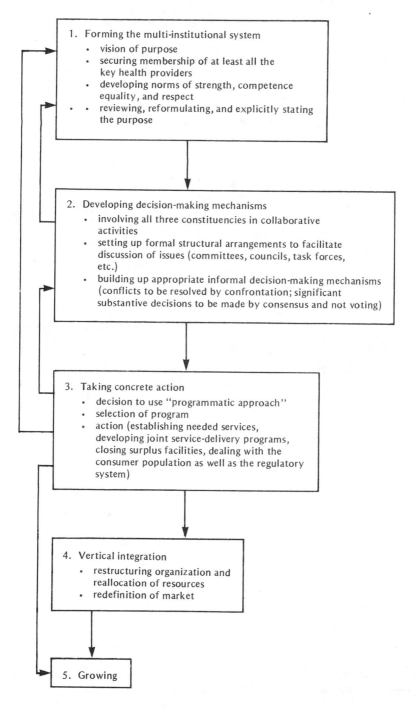

1. Forming the multi-institutional system
   - vision of purpose
   - securing membership of at least all the key health providers
   - developing norms of strength, competence equality, and respect
   - reviewing, reformulating, and explicitly stating the purpose

2. Developing decision-making mechanisms
   - involving all three constituencies in collaborative activities
   - setting up formal structural arrangements to facilitate discussion of issues (committees, councils, task forces, etc.)
   - building up appropriate informal decision-making mechanisms (conflicts to be resolved by confrontation; significant substantive decisions to be made by consensus and not voting)

3. Taking concrete action
   - decision to use "programmatic approach"
   - selection of program
   - action (establishing needed services, developing joint service-delivery programs, closing surplus facilities, dealing with the consumer population as well as the regulatory system)

4. Vertical integration
   - restructuring organization and reallocation of resources
   - redefinition of market

5. Growing

Chapter 10

Leadership

Managing collaboration and especially paradigmatic change requires skills and abilities over and above those of clinicians or
managers. This chapter describes case studies from which may be
gleaned some principles and generalizations. Once again an organizational change situation is described first, and then a selection of
collaborative situations are discussed.

Dr. V. is a psychiatrist who has guided a large psychiatric hospital
at Ermelo, Holland, from a traditional custodial care institution to a
modern mental health facility at the forefront of enlightened
psychiatric treatment. He is unusually perceptive about this process
and also about the long, difficult personal transition he made from
psychiatrist to manager.

His psychiatric hospital deals with a full range of mental disorders
serving a large community of 500,000, and providing a full range of
services. It is one of the largest psychiatric hospitals in Holland with
800 beds, 30 members on the medical staff, and a total of 802
staff—a patient-staff ratio of 1:1. This hospital belongs to a group of
six working together. In the whole country there are about thirty-
nine psychiatric hospitals, so this association is a big part of the total.

Portions of this chapter have appeared in "HMCR Interviews," in vol. 1, no. 1
and in vol. 2, no. 1, of the *Health Care Management Review*. Used with
permission of Aspen Systems Corporation, Germantown, Maryland.

Like many American hospitals, his contains largely semiprivate accommodations. It has many modern buildings, as well as restaurants, and playgrounds for children, lots of bright colors, good modern design, and attractive pictures that make the place look more like a well-designed recreation resort than a mental hospital.

On his arrival in 1963, the hospital had 860 beds and was seventy-five years old, with run-down buildings and locked, crowded wards. The hospital had a bad name not just in the neighborhood but also in the country. The admissions were low—about 250 a year at that time. The way people were handled was more or less cruel. There was much fighting. There was not very much variety in active treatment. The wards were dirty, and the smell was sometimes awful.

There were two initial tasks: first, to increase the number of personnel and to change their attitudes and, second, to change a lot of the buildings. The first goal of changing the people's attitudes—patients and personnel—could not be done without first changing the buildings so that people could imagine something else, could feel themselves in another environment.

Dr. V. did not work alone, but rather with the board of directors and the heads of several departments. His task was mostly to bring in new ideas. When they had agreed to them, then he carried them out.

The situation he found himself in was typically one of paradigmatic conflict in the sense that though the conditions were bad, no one wanted to change them except the board.

> I found it astonishing that nobody asked me to change things. The only people who asked me to change anything was the hospital board. In the hospital itself, I think the morale was so bad and so low that nobody had the inspiration or incentive to change. So in the first years, I had a lonely position because my ideas were not in equilibrium with the ideas of the others.

Or perhaps change was more threatening than the status quo. He could have used the power of the board to make unilateral changes, but:

> I felt it was important to involve the staff, to get them to work together. In the first few years they were advisory to me. I think that was because I was so impressed by the bad circumstances in the hospital that I had no time to think about new ways of cooperation, you know. So, my way of working was at that time to ask them if they agreed with what I thought. I was in a hurry to change circumstances and had the feeling of no support. Even the doctors were spectators instead of cooperators.

Dr. V.'s ideas and ideals certainly represented a new paradigm. He wanted to transform the old custodial authoritarian values, treatment, and organization into something with totally different goals, technology, organization and, above all, values:

> I thought that a mental hospital should be not a hospital alone, but a school for life where you can learn how to live. I thought the situation had to be friendly, open, nice. If people are anxious they need an environment where they feel at home. The second thing I tried to create was the situation in which the patient could participate in the treatment, where the treatment goals were based on learning principles. I thought it was important for them that they could learn to bargain with the doctors and psychologists about how their treatment should be done. I thought that it was important that they could speak about their problems, not only in a psychiatric way, but also in a human way, based on repair of relationships.

He did not find the task easy, nor did he at first approach it well, in relying on his traditional role of physician and authority.

> It was very depressing for me when I came to the hospital. Nobody—patients or staff—said anything about their personal problems to me. I was "The Boss," and they had to be very careful with me—they had the feeling it could be dangerous or something!
>
> You know, I made a mistake in the first few years. Not only because I was in a hurry to change things, but also because I had no idea, no clear idea, about the directorship. I mean, I knew clearly what I wanted to do—that was no problem—but at that time I was more a doctor than a director. I thought that if you prescribé things, everybody does it. If you prescribe a medicine, a treatment, as a doctor you think that everybody listens. I would issue orders and then find out that nothing happened.
>
> Of course I was if I expressed my anger it would not help very much. I had no idea what to do. At first I thought the best thing to do was to leave. I felt that if I were such a bad director that nobody listened to me, I would do better to leave.

This precipitated his own personal crisis of change.

> I did a lot of thinking about it. Why didn't I leave? I do not know exactly, but I think I believed that it could be done, that I needed more time, and that I was another person than everybody believed I was.
>
> A lot of people said to me at that time, "You are for me the fourth director. And everything will stay the same." I began to realize very deeply that without the cooperation of the staff, the work could not be done. So I tried to find new ways of cooperation. I brought people together; we tried to speak together in groups, in small groups or bigger ones. I organized groups of different kinds of people and tried to find common

ideas with them. It was very hesitant in the beginning, of course. They were very careful; they were not clear, but I got the idea that more or less they accepted me.

How did he change?

I think that I did not attack them anymore. I tried to understand the situation they were in, in that they tried to do things well as they saw it. They did not mean to do things incorrectly, but it was because they did not see, at that moment, what I thought I saw. I lost my earlier professional way of prescribing things. I think that was the change in myself.

This change took some three or four years. But the fuller appreciation of the new roles needed took longer:

I thought we needed not only groups of people working together, but also to have those groups working in such a way that the goal of the hospital could be attained. You remember the goal I mentioned before—being a school for life. But nobody in the hospital, including myself, had any idea of what kind of organization we needed. We were all professionals. To be an "organization man or woman" asked another attitude, another role, another way of thinking. We all needed to learn this new role.

This took, in all, about seven years. It required not only Dr. V.'s persistence, but bringing people in from the outside. There was not very much resistance in the nursing staff, but in the medical staff there was a lot of resistance. They were the most powerful in the hospital, and they were anxious about the nursing staff growing in power. He introduced investigators from the outside to both the nursing staff and the medical staff, and the medical staff felt that only they should have been involved. So they were angry.

He thought that the best thing to do was to start with the nursing staff and that the interest of the medical staff would grow, then as things developed, he would involve them in the whole process more intensively.

The first thing we needed was to get a clear motivation to change, and to learn to work together in an organization. So I hired two people, a sociologist and an organization consultant, who investigated several groups in the hospital. I asked them to find out what people thought about the way we were working together in the hospital. That was the starting point. I promised that everything that was said in the groups was secret, so everybody could say what he liked. The director could only get information if a group wished to give it. That gave a lot of motivation because everybody could say what they liked without a feeling of danger for themselves.

What was interesting and difficult was the fact that once again all the groups were very critical of me. Since people have a lot of difficulties among themselves, it is a normal process for them to need to speak out about their anxieties and difficulties with each other before they can work together. The first thing they need to do is to tell them to the director or the leader. I suppose they need to discover "will he punish me or not?" For the leader it is very difficult, I think, because I was doing something well; I am trying to cooperate with my people—and in the first meetings you find the contrary.

The investigators helped him a lot to deal with this seeming ingratitude. The process of redefinition continued slowly.

We tried to find out about the new roles. We spoke first about the uneasy feelings we had for each other, and then we spoke about our new roles and the contents of them—about the role of a director, what people expect from me, and what I expect from my people. I talked with all my department heads about it, and they spoke with their co-workers. So we found out new ways of cooperation, new attitudes, and new organization models.

New attitudes often means new people. There were many new people. Every year they brought in thirty or forty new people. But these were replacements for normal attrition and few, all because of the changes. In the medical staff practically nobody left; in fact, it was growing every year by two or three people. Now there are thirty members of the medical staff where they started with only five.

Things changed not only for patients, but staff: a school for learning was both.

We said that promotion is not the only goal in life. We introduced a learning philosophy that we call "permanent education." If you get promoted, it is nice, but it is not the only important goal. We said that what is most important is to grow personally, to develop yourself. Therefore, permanent education is a very important issue now. A lot of people are following courses, and are trying to develop themselves either professionally or managerially.

Ironically, this growth means an acceptance of turnover since they do not have all kinds of higher jobs in the hospital and therefore a lot a people might like to leave in the next few years.

The process graphically described involved both attitude and concrete change. Slow and painful, the transformation still continues. A crucial juncture was the appreciation of Dr. V. of the world of those he wished to change, a grudging respect was essential for them in turn to begin to trust him and the process in which he engaged them.

Turning now to some examples from collaborative endeavors, first to be considered are two contrasting approaches to merger, which raise questions about how far and how fast, as well as issues of style, especially participative involvement versus authoritarian change. Then the former executive vice-president of Affiliated Hospitals and John Danielson of Capital Area Health Consortium reflect on their jobs.

> "I'm still amazed that I was able to do it the way I did," said Dr. E. as he reflected upon his experiences gained during a merger several years ago. "I acted like a bull in a china shop. I would never do it in the same way again. All the same, it worked. Probably because I arranged to clear up the whole business in one year and then leave. For this reason, those involved more or less accepted what was done. Occasionally they expressed their negative feelings, but on the whole they kept them to themselves. I was to be succeeded by someone else and they only had to accept me temporarily. Fortunately for them, and also for me. I did not have to worry about it too much, as I had agreed, in the interests of the merger, to stay for one year and no longer.

Dr. E. hit on the idea of a one-year stint after having heard a great deal about similar situations in industry where mergers are often brought about under temporary management. He knew little about merger problems, especially the human side. He had been a general practitioner for fifteen years before becoming director of a hospital and was faced with the problems without any previous knowledge.

Why did he take it on? He thought that two hospitals in close proximity to one another in a small provincial town should combine forces. In this way a greatly improved service could be offered to the area. Second, he enjoyed challenges.

> I like doing difficult things. I think that I need them. Being director is not interesting enough when it only concerns settling all sorts of matters which one is faced with every day and which requires a solution. Occasionally one must be able to accomplish something which at first sight seemed almost impossible. I enjoy such problems and if I tackle something I am prepared, if necessary, to struggle through to the end, through thick and thin. I have already said that with the experience I now have, I probably would not dare to do that again, but I would do it with the same tenacity. That is part of me, I think, also part of my strength.

The action took place in a small provincial town where there were two hospitals. One was Catholic with 147 beds, the other Protestant with 137 beds. Most of the specialists, with the exception of the specialists for internal medicine, worked in both hospitals. The hospital with 147 beds had a specialist for internal medicine as medical director who, it was rumored, had failed to obtain a professorship. Dr. E. was the medical director of the other hospital. His hospital had a number of problems. Too few beds were occupied, there were solvency difficulties, staffing was not ideal, the quality of work was poor, and there was no radiologist.

He felt something should be done, especially when it became evident that new buildings were necessary. He sent a note to the board of trustees in which he expressed the urgent wish for a merger with the other hospital that had a whole wing lying empty. This resulted in a secret meeting between the boards of trustees of both hospitals, but nothing came of it. He then deliberately let the news of the note leak out in order to precipitate a discussion. It was soon evident that almost all the specialists were in favor of a merger. Only the specialists for internal medicine held back. The boards of trustees then publicly resumed their discussions. They were unable to reach agreement alone, but with some outside consulting help, they succeeded.

He was asked to actually arrange the merger and to do it in such a way that all beds were to be contained in the larger hospital that had become much too big since the recent construction of additional buildings. There were several possibilities open, bearing in mind that both hospitals were severely understaffed and therefore much too empty. The number of beds was finally fixed at 220.

Within several weeks of officially taking up his position as merger director, he ordered several departments to be moved. No one was given a say in the matter. Those involved were told to move, and that had to suffice. The specialists had declared themselves in favor, and that simplified matters. The specialists for internal medicine finally succumbed when it became evident that the process could not be arrested any longer.

As always with a merger, new functions were created. People became subordinate to former equals, and departments were amalgamated. That this caused dissatisfaction became noticeable from reduced numbers and absenteeism through illness.

I did not worry too much about this as I would be leaving anyway. I did not feel personally involved and this aloofness made it possible to act firmly, sometimes perhaps even harshly. People were, however, allowed to express their opinions, not in connection with the merger, but about a new hospital to be built in the future. Everyone was asked to think about the requirements for the new building.

It was all settled within a year. One organization in one building with one management. The determination to succeed made accomplishment possible.

> "I repeat," said Dr. E., "only now do I see clearly the problems which I overlooked. All the same, it is satisfying to see, now eight years later, the contours of a new hospital rising from the ground. By the way, I should also mention that I did have some difficulty in finding a new job as medical director. Evidently the methods which I employed do not earn one a good name. Fortunately it did not take long, after having been snubbed a few times, before I once again took up the appointment as medical director in a large hospital."

This story contrasts sharply with the next vignette.

Ten years ago in a medium-sized town, there were two hospitals, one Catholic with 346 beds and the other Protestant with 250 beds. The Catholic hospital, in particular, was in need of new buildings. The Protestant one was comparatively new.

The administrator at the Catholic hospital, Mr. O., who at that time had just joined the hospital, was strongly in favor of a merger because new additional buildings would be feasible and of use only if both hospitals were to join forces.

Mr. O. had studied economics in his spare time. Before joining the hospital, he had spent twenty years in industry, in marketing. He had been involved in two large mergers and was especially aware of the human problems of such situations. He deliberately chose to enter the health sector. He was socially conscious and felt unable to develop sufficiently in industry where commerce was too dominant for his taste. He enjoyed fighting for his ideals and was fascinated by people. In 1976 he obtained a master's degree in marketing. In his job he tried to work from two basic principles:

> To remain faithful to one's own discipline, in this case the economy. That means that in daily practice I try to gather figures and other possible information and present them to people who can help and convince in the formulation and possible putting into effect of management policies.
>
> To remain oneself as much as possible as a human being with both one's strong and weak qualities. Also to strive towards good human relation-

ships. To be a sort of leaven. Tenacious and presevering where it seems necessary.

Mr. O. could lose his temper and could not abide gossips, whom he shut up. Because of his career in industry he felt that he understood the employee's way of thinking. He tolerated straightforward opposition fairly well. He had learned to cope with feelings, such as frustration, from experience, but coping remained difficult for him, and it was not always possible to answer or do as he would wish. He believed that tenacity coupled with flexibility were important and that if a leader set about his business systematically and democratically, his fellow workers would follow suit.

Initially, both boards of trustees, and in particular, the chairmen, were of the opinion that cooperation should evolve without commitment. Mutual information would be provided, but each party would be able to go its own way. Mr. O. advised going to a consulting firm because he felt that a merger should be made. The consultants came to the same conclusion. The advice was to amalgamate into one organization with two establishments, with one board and one management. The thirty to forty members of the medical staff, most of whom worked in both hospitals, also advised merging into one hospital. That, however, was not then feasible.

Initially, the boards stood by their view of loose cooperation. Mr. O. made sure that they were regularly provided with information on population figures and market research as a basis from which they would gradually be able to form the opinion that a merger was better. The atmosphere in which discussions were held remained relaxed, partly due to the clarity of the information. However, it took a great deal of time, in fact three years, to decide on a merger.

Mr. O. then began a process that led to the centralization of some nonclinical services, namely, administration, personnel, and technical services. They all moved to one building in the grounds of the Protestant hospital. The process began with the making of comparable estimates and continued from there. One administrator left. One purchasing manager was appointed for the totality. Several people retired, including a medical director and a matron, and the administrator of the other hospital was assigned to Mr. O. as an assistant, by mutual agreement. Gradually matters developed so that there was one training school and one medical team. The subspecialists shifted to one hospital, with internal medicine and surgery in the other.

The whole process went on for six years. Eventually it was hoped to merge into one hospital, but that would take some time yet. Mr. O. was amazed that the amalgamation of management services went so smoothly. He thought that the reason for this was that it did not have to be done in too much of a hurry because those involved were allowed to participate fully in making the decision. Above all, the objectives of the merger were clear.

It would still be many years yet before all employees were installed in one new hospital. Mr. O. had, however, bearing in mind his experience in the matter so far, very high expectations of this event.

The issues contrasted here are not simply resolved. The painstaking involvement of Mr. O. seems more human and less disruptive than Dr. E.'s impetuousness. Yet delay costs, in money and pain. The longer uncertainty endures, the more people suffer. How long? Perhaps there is no clear answer, except that of "timing, timing and timing," as Mr. W. of Affiliated Hospitals would have it.

> If anybody knew how to tell you what the right time was, he'd have the answer to all kinds of questions. Some fellow said there are three criteria for buying real estate: location, location and location. We convert that and say there are three major things we regard in administration: timing, timing and timing. It's a judgment call. If it gets out too soon, you blow your cover and you get a lot of people offended about it. But there will come a time probably when they will want to keep it quiet and you're better off to let it leak, because if the millieu is conducive to it, then the fact that it's being discussed brings pressure to bear on whoever is doing the negotiating to produce something, either do it or not do it.

January 1, 1975, marked the merger, after 15 years of discussion and negotiation, of the Peter Bent Brigham Hospital, the Boston Hospital for Women, and the Robert B. Brigham Hospital into the Affiliated Hospitals Center. Mr. W.'s job was as executive vice-president, to supervise the planning for the 680-bed Affiliated Hospitals Center that was to replace the facilities of all three hospitals.

He also shares Mr. O.'s concern with creating credibility but feels it may often have to be done by an outside character. This reflects the proposition, put forward earlier, that the uninvolved visionary above the fray is critical to paradigmatic change.

> The common rule is that main negotiators in the merger have got to be a small group of key trustees who are prepared to see it happen. Let me put it this way. In merger negotiations I think there needs to be a figure who has enormous credibility. By credibility I simply mean that people tend to believe that if he's for it, it must be good and that he's not out to feather his own nest. The paid people always have an axe to grind and even if they

succeed in rising above that, nobody will believe them. Ok? So the paid people are not credible activists in the negotiating process except behind the scenes. The only exception is a situation where a small hospital is merging with a large one. In that case sometimes the administrator of the larger one can be that figure. But usually you will have two main actors, one from each board. Sometimes it will be a grand old man, somebody let's say who is 68 years old, who maybe would announce in advance that he or she will not take a seat on the new board, and who thereby establishes credibility in the situation to be able to deal with everybody. But failing that, then I think a midwife is a good thing to look for. Sometimes it can be an attorney, sometimes a consultant.

Mr. W. is very explicit on the need, as stated previously in relation to the Newbury merger, to manage the collaborative process: It just does not happen of its own accord.

I suppose the thing that is special about handling a hospital merger is that you have what is essentially a voluntary environment. That is to say, you are really in a situation where the parties cannot be compelled to do anything. Whereas in the ordinary bureaucracy you have got some kind of sanctions that you can impose. You give somebody a raise or you do not give them a raise, or you promote somebody or you do not promote them, or if they have a request you can approve it or disapprove it. Those kinds of sanctions are not available to you in a merging situation. What is available to you in a merging situation is more in the class of political sanctions, which was best summarized when The Godfather talked about making people "offers they could not refuse." In other words, what you have to do is to think in terms of how can you create a situation so that behavior oriented toward your objective of merger is, if not more rewarding, at least less problematic than behavior in the opposite direction.

What you would need at that point is to draw on some understanding about board members, what their motivations are and what drummer they march to, right? I for one work on the assumption that they are volunteers, so they are not in it for money, but it is a position of community leadership and what they aspire to in effect is the respect of their "community." Our term for it down here is "conversations at lunch on State Street." State Street is sort of a symbol of the Boston downtown, a high powered community, and those guys down there have lunch, and that is a little mini-public. For them it represents public opinion. Those people tend to be pretty political themselves. They understand the ambitions, and they talk, and there are fads that go around and they gossip like anybody else. And most of those guys down there want to be thought of as being with it. All right?

Mr. W. is particularly clear and helpful on the distinction between political (with a small *p*) behavior and manipulation.

Effective institutional administration requires a lot more of this kind of political behavior than is commonly talked about. There is a general social tendency to avoid thinking that we have to do things in a political way. People think that political implies a devious, contrived, self-serving kind of manipulated behavior. But everyone is political; you know, somebody said life is a political experience from the first time you play your mother off against your father over when to go to bed. That is a political maneuver, but our culture does not like to think ithose terms, and people would be very uncomfortable if I said, "well now, let me tell you what I really did, you know I maneuvered this guy into a box, right, and he could not get out of it because he did not have any choice." That just does not sound nice.

I have always felt that if you manipulate to impose your will or to enhance your own position, that would be immoral. But what you have in these situations is a general goal on which there is a broad consensus; it is just that everybody sees it a little differently and each person has his own interests or responsibilities to protect. What you have to do is to manage things so that the goal is achieved, but in a way everybody can live with, even though nobody gets everything he wants. Now you have to remember that every one of those people has a duty to look after his own thing, that all the others are doing that too, and you cannot get where they want to go unless all of that gets worked out. In my experience, they do not mind so long as everybody plays fair and there is confidence that it is being done in the interest of the big goal.

Viewing the dynamics of a merger as a set of social pressures you can guide, is the most productive approach. If you are trying to quarterback this thing, the main thing to recognize is that merger is not happening because you willed. The merger is happening because there are a lot of planets out there with the right alignment. If you stay out of their way and just nudge them, you get your results. If the planets are not in their right alignment, you might as well forget it—it is not going to happen, at least if they are so far out of alignment that even with a little nudge from you they will not get in.

The approach to a merger I am suggesting is not passive, although I do not have a Captain-on-the Bridge kind of style, partly because I do not think I would be any good at it and maybe because of that I rationalize that I do not think it is any good. I would characterize my management style as reactive management and a style of reacting to pressures. Now if you want to do that well, if you want to get somewhere, then you have to influence the pressures to which you are going to react—ok?

Manage the problems, the pain, and the conditions for solution. Mr. W., however, does agree with Dr. E. about the value of a timetable for creating a sense of urgency.

Another thing that creates pressures to act are deadlines. Around the flimsiest kind of rationale you can often get a date set and a deadline established, and that deadline should not be too far out there because that just improves geometrically the chances of something coming up that would bollix it up. So you have a short deadline, you can reduce the risk of unanticipated events and you keep everybody's nose right hard against those deadlines.

In our merger we just laid out a timetable and it was the tightest timetable we could put together. If everybody did not do what they had to do at precisely the right date, we were going to miss it. The key to it was that every hospital membership, which is hordes of people, had to vote by two thirds and they had to have a 30 day notice for the meeting. Fortunately the Lord was with us, and one of the board presidents picked it up and said, "Well, we will do it at our annual meeting in November," and the idea that they would do it at their annual meeting grabbed hold, and then someone said, "why not?" They were the ones with the largest number of members, a couple of hundred, so they had to get proxies and the merger agreement out to all those people. When they went out I said, "now it is over. It is done." Because having sent that out to 200 people in town, thereby saying, "this is it, we are going to do it," then failing to deliver on that, everybody would be embarrassed out of his mind.

I mean if we lost the election, that would be one thing; but the failure on everybody else's part to follow through, recommend it and try to get the proxies in and all that, would make everyone look like asses. Well there was a fair amount of screaming and yelling after that, but nobody wanted to be the one to hold it up. And my concern was that I not do something dumb. I had more potential to mess it up than I did to enhance it at that point because the procedure was rolling.

Returning to credibility, like Dr. V., he has worked hard to earn it.

The more open you can be, the better, in my judgment. You have to recognize in a situation like ours that the actors are all able people and they have their strengths too. I do not believe in taking advantage of people. I think that if one of the people out there is working under some kind of handicap because he does not have some critical information or something, then I have an obligation not to capitalize on that. That is partly a moral point, but it is practical too—if you win on that basis it always comes back to haunt you later. But most of the people were perfectly able to take care of themselves and they just counted on us to be up to playing our part. In fact, they would have been insulted, and rightly so, if we had proceeded on the assumption they had to be nursemaided. In that kind of situation, the more disclosure of strategy the better because if everybody is trying to get to the same place, it will help and if not, then there is no way to do it with secret strategy. Besides, they would figure it out anyway and think you were just trying to be cute or, as the British would say, too clever by half.

What all of this requires is credibility and confidence. People really have to believe that you are being fair and that what you are after is a solution that benefits everybody as much as it can. Let me give you an example of something that happened after the merger. I had agreed to work up a report that showed that everybody was being treated fairly on a particular subject. In a meeting I was getting pressure to get the report out, and I finally confessed that I was procrastinating because I was not sure everybody could live with the results. One of the people said, "hell, you built a career on making the facts fit the conclusion." Everybody had a big laugh and we went on to the next agenda item.

Well, I took that as a compliment. I got the message that everybody knew there was no good answer and that what was needed was something that moved the project along in a way that everybody could live with. In other words, they believed I would not use the report to stir things up, but to solve problems if I could, and that if I had to gloss something over or strain an interpretation, it would be in the interests of trying to get the thing settled.

Assuming my interpretation was right, it is evidence of the kind of credibility you work hard to earn. You do not get it overnight, and in order to keep it you keep working at it. Sometimes you do something that loses some of it and then you have to work overtime to get it back.

I sometimes tell young administrators that when you are given a job, the trustees put a hundred dollars worth of confidence in your account. When you handle a tough situation well, they put a couple more dollars in, and when you blow one they take a batch out. You cannot let the balance get to zero because then you are through even if they do not fire you.

An interesting issue is whether to reduce uncertainty by crystallizing outcome such as being clear as to future structures (and who will occupy what jobs) in order to reduce pain, or whether this will increase resistance. Mr. W. believes it will.

My basic rule is to keep the issues to a minimum. The point of the merger strategy is to create something that is conducive to agreement and obviously the more issues you inject into it, the less your chance for arriving at agreement, right? Now there are certain minimal things you have to do as required by law. You have to have bylaws for the surviving corporation and you have to know who the new board is going to be. Practically speaking, there are at least one or two other things you need to get settled, particularly who the chief executive is going to be—it makes you nervous if you sit on the board and the day after the merger you do not know who is in charge of the place.

But you should try desperately to avoid deciding questions like how exactly you are going to merge services or who is going to be the director of what. You have the almost physical problem of getting them settled at the same time because you get one thing settled and by the time you have got another thing settled, the first one has come unglued. The other thing is, everyone who is settled alienates somebody, so you have the problem of losing support every time you settle something. We call it the principle of the omnibus bill; you put 40 issues in a piece of legislation and any one of might pass, but the accumulated opposition to all 40 of them is enough to kill the whole bill.

He summarizes his style in the following words:

Now the style that I described to you pays a lot of attention to emotional factors and sensibilities, and I think that behavior of that sort is conducive to the merger process. It is a massage thing, a kind of orchestration of forces, a not being front and center unless you have to. I want to say one other thing about that style though, it is not a substitute for toughness.

There is a time when you can sense that the level of frustration is at a point where what is called for is a strong move, even one that may hurt somebody. If you set all these forces in motion and then are not prepared to pay the price when the day comes of disabusing somebody of what he thought he was going to get, then you just end up with mass confusion. Do not misunderstand. Toughness has got two components, I think. One is the guts to do it. A lot of people have guts. And the other thing is to do it at a time and way that gets the job done. Ok? There is no point in going out there and showing them how big your gun is if there is not anything in front of it. A lot of misapprehension about management style is that people say, "he has got a lot of guts, but he does not know when to use them."

The disconcerting thing about toughness is that oftentimes when you display it you upset a lot of people; well, what should I say, upset, that is the right word, but not enough, they are dismayed, they sort of stand there with their mouths open and they have been through all of this gentle business and everybody has gotten used to the gentle approach and then all of a sudden bang. And then people say, "boy, I did not expect that," and you feel it is unfair because they were caught unawares, and you do a lot of talking to yourself. That is one of the things that is left out of most of the discussions about participative management, that it actually can create greater concentrations of power than the other kind because people in cooperative work situations become extremely dependent on whoever is playing the leadership role. It can get to be an unhealthy paternalistic situation if you are not careful. In rigid, authoritarian, autocratic systems you think he is a sonofabitch, but he is the vice president and I will put up with him, right? And I owe him so much for my salary and that by God is what he will get and that is all. That is an element of personal independence that tends to disappear in the participative system, so you know, you do not get anything for nothing.

I think the style I am talking about is suited to the kind of thing I get paid to do, to help formulate policies and direction, to develop people internally and maintain an environment for strong cohesive programs. But it is no way to fight a naval engagement; it is no way to run an operating room, and I do not think it is a good way to run a laundry business. I think production and functioning people have to do what they are told, and there is no point in being manipulative. Sure, every office has politics and you can use some of that to maintain peace and morale, but I do not think a straightforward sort of production-oriented operating function calls for a participative style.

John Danielson, in his tenure now completed at the Capital Area Health Consortium, also regarded credibility as crucial, not simply to himself, but among the participants in the collaborative process.

He has explicitly tried to create an atmosphere of trust among the consortium members.

We approach problems so that no one is going to be badly hurt. If somebody is bleeding, we all go to help that person, rather than to encourage the basic human animal instinct to kill a bleeding and wounded tiger. You do not need a wounded tiger in the bush. You either kill him or cure him, but do not leave him there. We try to help somebody who is in trouble because someone in trouble is going to be a problem and a real difficulty to the system. And it is my job to try and convince them of that and keep them talking together. It is an extraordinarily difficult thing to do.

Danielson functioned as a personal consultant. He knew the members personally, and therefore they trusted him to interpret for them when something was going wrong, so he could steer them back to the right track. But most of all, he kept them from killing each other.

Most hospital administrators do not understand that the real issue is the management of patient care, and that is why I am involved in what I am doing here. The issue here is the management of patient care. It is not the management of things. I view the institutions as they were biological entities. They ingest, digest, excrete, throw up, get sick, have personalities, get nervous, they are suspicious, they are competitive, they are everything. Each institution is a biological entity; it has a clear characteristic personality, and what it does is never accidental. It has always got a reason. It is my job to know what the reason is. It is the same with people, so I regard them as people. I do not see 3800 beds in front of me at the board meetings, I see nine people.

He describes his role as executive director as follows:

My job is neither to control the members personally or to run their affairs, but is to be able to put those tigers on the stools so the act will be performed, and when a tiger is off the stool, I have to find him and get him back on the stool, or the people will want their money back. I do not jump through the hoops and I do not do the performance. All I am in there for is to make sure that everybody else does their thing successfully so we all come out of it okay.

He saw himself as a "facilitator," the person who helped the group know when they had reached a consensus.

We can get consensus prospectively or we can get consensus retrospectively, It does not make any difference. If we get consensus retrospectively, what we have done is a beautiful thing. It tells everybody what we did and why. Now if we were wrong and could not get consensus retrospectively, we would all agree to help figure out some way to deal with what had been done. Everybody is going to make mistakes. All we have to agree to is to put the issue on the table. We start talking about it and agree that no one will act until the group has been brought to a consensus. That is my job.

There were times when the consensus approach would not work. One was when there was not enough time. The consortium was never meant to constipate the institutions and be another authority. It was meant to be a facilitator and was supposed to make their job easier, quicker, and better so that they could be in charge of their own strategy and could take the intent of Congress and meet it, but bend the regulations. No one would ever hold them to be irresponsible if they bent the regulations but fulfilled the intent of Congress.

The second time the consensus approach would not work was if the consortium had 50 percent of the cards, and the feds or the HSA or somebody in authority held the other hand. If they were told that they could have only one cardiac surgery program in Hartford, then since both St. Francis Hospital and Hartford Hospital have cardiac surgery programs, talking for a thousand years would never result in consensus.

What happened in this situation is that they began to review the options:

That is my job, to help those two institutions come up with alternatives. It is very important not to just accept what somebody says, but to examine the reasons why there only ought to be one cardiac surgery program in Hartford. After quite a bit of deliberation, they decided to keep both heart surgery programs, since the capital investment was already there, and move the team instead of the people. Why move the patients if you can move the team? They joined the two heart surgery teams together into one and began to operate in both places.

He admitted that the members came up with that alternative:

With a little help. Somebody has got to help them. There has always got to be somebody around to help them.

He believed that an executive director should not be hired for a consortium board until the "process" had been decided upon. Once this had occurred, the implementation of the process should become the job of the executive director. He suggested that there were four loyalties that were constant companions to the board members:

First is the loyalty to their own hospital. Second is the loyalty to the profession that they represent, or their ethic and its effort. The third is the loyalty to the patient and to the community. the fourth is the loyalty to the Consortium. It is my job to make sure that the loyalty to this Consortium is not in conflict with the other three.

One of the most difficult things he had to contend with was keeping a "low profile," and getting the members to understand that the consortium was theirs, not his.

For those who were interested in becoming an executive director of a consortium, he gave the following advice:

Somebody once asked me what kind of a textbook I would recommend for reading material, and I said, "there is only one, and that is the Bible." Read the Bible and you will know how to run a consortium. It is all there.

His comments echo those of Dr. V. Trust, respect, facilitation, and help he offered and offered in an unassuming way. His roles were defined by an admiring trustee: facilitator, planner, peacemaker, diplomat, politician, public relations, elder statesman. Note the emphasis again on politician with a small *p*.

Finally a summary of leadership skills as reflected in the varying need for different skills at the different stages of the collaborative process: political arbitration is a key skill that multi-institutional leaders—both outsiders (e.g., the executive director of the consortium) and insiders (e.g., the key leaders of the member institutions)—must bring to use during stage 1, the formative period in the evolution of collaborative systems. Leaders of individual institutions may have to make decisions that involve conflict of interest. Unless they have given thought to the problem of dual roles and have established relationships of trust and power with their own constituencies at home, the multi-institutional system will begin to crumble.

Formal decision-making mechanisms, however, need always to be complemented with appropriate informal decision-making mechanisms. The main consideration in this particular situation is that multi-institutional leadership has very little formal authority over the individual organizations. Thus not only does information have to be provided on its own initiative, the implementation of any resulting decisions is also very often voluntary. Therefore, in situations with high existing conflict, the possibility exists that the information provided by organizations may be incomplete, biased, or deliberately false; further, it may be difficult to arrive at joint decisions; and, once joint decisions have been arrived at, implementation may not always take place according to plan. The task of the interorganizational leaders in such a case becomes that of creating a situation in which (a) members provide valid information in the joint decision-making arena, (b) they have free choice in agreeing/disagreeing over a decision, so that (c) they develop internal commitments to the decisions that are finally made; this would also ensure a high likelihood that the decisions would be implemented.

In stage 2—the developing of appropriate decision-making mechanisms—the crucial leadership skills are those of "process facilitation." In the Capital Area Health Consortium, a more successful health consortium, the key multi-institutional leader, the executive director, had substantial experience as a competent facilitator, and among other things had instituted the informal norms that (a) conflicts would be resolved by confrontation and not by smoothing over or forcing decisions through, and (b) all key substantive decisions would be made by consensus, and not by voting.

The crucial leadership skills needed at stage 3 are those that promote courage, trust, and a resolution among the consortium members to stick by earlier commitments and a grasp of incentive systems.

The fourth stage is paradigmatic—the irreversible shifts in resources and structure must be brought off. Credibility and "above the fray" are crucial. Understanding the paradigmatic nature of the process, and worlds are finally in conflict, worlds that cannot understand each other, is eseential if success is to be forthcoming. Stage 5 requires little new in the way of leadership skills.

Collaborative leadership, as the move toward some type of regional health system quickens, is thus a quantum leap different from institutional leadership. More statesmanlike in nature, it requires a Janus-like ability to face in and out simultaneously; to see the world of the institution as it sees it, as well as the larger world outside. It is, after all, the thesis of this book that true and significant collaboration involves a change in world and world views, a paradigm shift. The paradox of passionate vision, with no axe to grind (to mix metaphors) seems essential. However, realism must temper even the most capable executive. It would seem that collaboration will be trivial and relatively peripheral in nature in most instances, and that many structural forms now popular are essentially unstable. The fashion for falling in step must give place to a more sanguine assessment of what does and can work and when nothing will, rather than an adherence to ideas, however appealing. The retention of a vision of what can be, rooted in the reality of what is, and a knowledge of how to get there, is perhaps after all the true measure of leadership.

Index

About the Author

Alan Sheldon is Associate Professor and Director of Executive Programs at the Harvard School of Public Health. He trained as a physician and psychiatrist at Cambridge University and Westminster Hospital in England before becoming involved in management education at Harvard Business School, where he headed the first-year organizational behavior course in the M.B.A. program. Dr. Sheldon's research interests include leadership and the management of planning and of collaboration. He consults widely in both the private and public sectors, specializing in the health field and public broadcasting. He is the author of over a dozen books and seventy articles.